Heal Yourself
And Stay Healthy!

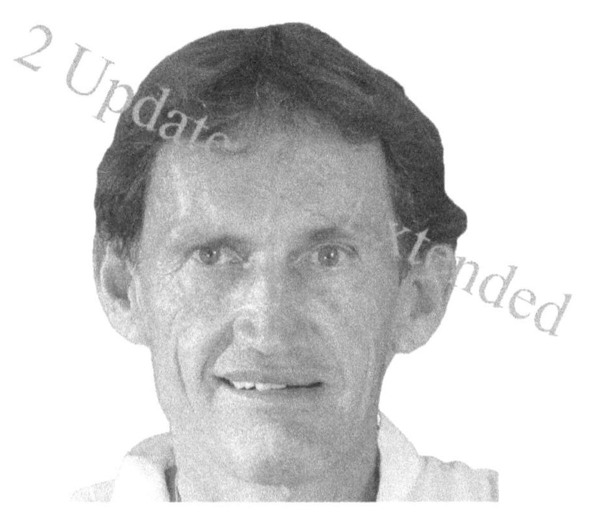

Learn The Cause Of Diseases
- psychosomatic or weak immune system-

And How To Heal Diabetes,

Cancer, Heart, Back…

Health and Fitness Expert
Rudi Zimmerer

Heal Yourself
And Stay Healthy!

Learn the cause of diseases - psychosomatic or weak immune system-
and how to heal diabetes, cancer,
heart, back…

Health and Fitness Expert
Rudi Zimmerer

Copyright © Rudi Zimmerer 2st edition,

Jul 2021 2Update and Extended.

Author: Rudi Zimmerer
Title: Heal Yourself And Stay Healthy
Sub: Learn the cause of diseases - psychosomatic or weak immune system-
and how to heal diabetes, cancer, heart, back…

ISBN-13: 9798539663315
Category: BODY, MIND & SPIRIT/Inspiration & Personal Growth

Publisher:
Rudolf Zimmerer

NOTE TO READERS

This publication contains the opinions and ideas of its author. It is intended to provide helpful and informative material on the subject addressed. The strategies/information outlined in
this book may not be suitable for everybody and are not guaranteed or warranted to produce any particular results.

This book is sold with the understanding that neither the author nor the publisher is engaged in rendering psychology, religious, medical or any other advice. The reader should consult a competent professional before adopting any of the suggestions in this book or drawing inferences from it.

No warranty is made with respect to the accuracy, authenticity or completeness of the information or references contained herein, and both the author and the publisher specifically disclaim any responsibility for any liability, loss or risk, personal or otherwise, which is incurred as a consequence, directly or indirectly, of the use and application of any of the contents of this book.

About the Author

Imagine my situation: I was a 22-year-old student studying electrical engineering, and I was involved in a major struggle with my professors because I had won the case against one of them to undo my last examination. All of the professors were very upset with me over this and gave me a hard time. Also, I was the founder of a new political party that won the last election of the student parliament. Also, I had epilepsy, the left side of my face was paralyzed, and I had many other diseases related to the stress. I was quite ill.

One beautiful Sunday, I went to the emergency doctor to receive my daily injection of Reparil. A very young, overtired doctor assisted me. While he was attempting to open the ampule, it broke. This made me nervous. He opened two new ampules and had to mix the contents of the two together. His hands were shaking, and he spilled one-third of the solution from one ampule onto the floor. I was scared and knew that it was possible to die if the injection was given incorrectly.

Nevertheless, he managed to fill the syringe. He tried to inject the medication into my vein but missed, then he tried it again and again. I became furious and protested against his treatment. Suddenly, he injected the solution
 into my vein very fast. I lost consciousness, saw my life passing by in colorful slides, and then I saw my body from the perspective of a fly on the ceiling. I was clinically dead.

I remembered my life up to that point. I had lived a life full of sorrow; I was abused and beaten by my family nearly every day. When I left the house to go to school, older and stronger children in the neighborhood would beat me up because my family was atheist. I could hardly learn my mother tongue, German, and I was a stutterer because my parents beat me for every mistake that I made, even when

I was innocent. Therefore, I went to a low-grade school and struggled to learn any languages.

At age sixteen, I'd apprenticed as a telecommunications installer and worked hard for twelve hours a day. I struggled with my boss because they were unjust, which I could not stand without protesting like crazy. I was scared to approach girls. My parents complained about me and always said, 'You are stupid and lazy'.

I started with positive thinking, autogenic training, and self-conditioning of my mind. The side effect was epilepsy. I complained all the time and was on the edge of suicide nearly every day. Nevertheless, I had one goal as a child: To become an engineer. I went to school again but failed in the first examination, so I had to take an additional oral examination in four subjects. I finally passed as a D student. I could then study at a university.

When the doctors revived me, I knew that the way I was living was entirely wrong, because I did not enjoy my life. Then I chose for my life to equal the sum of all my happiness.

I finished my studies as an A student in Dusseldorf, and with the support of the government, I did my advanced studies in Bremen far away from my parents. Still, I was depressed and desired to change my life, so I started to study, in addition to engineering, psychology. After some time, I started going to self-experience groups. Unfortunately, these groups were not much help, so I tried body-and-feelings-oriented therapy, combined with meditation.

When I was 26, I worked as an engineer and designed the navigation control unit for a satellite. My girlfriend was pregnant, but we lost the child. That was one of the worst setbacks and tragedies of my life, and also the springboard to God. While other people
might sink into depression after going through such a disaster, the opposite became real for me.

We all go through nightmares, but please don't remain stuck in them. Keep going!

Within two and a half years of starting the body-and-feelings- oriented therapy, I was able to escape my sorrow and become healthy.

In 2004, I was forced to leave the ashram due to an accident in Cologne on the Europe tour for Mata Amritanandamayi. I helped a woman to catch her train in the morning, and then I fell down on the pedestrian border. I felt this massive pain in my shoulder, people were coming to help me and wanted to bring me to the hospital, but I refused, because I had to return my rented car to Bremen (300km distance). During the night, I decided to go to the doctor, he gave me an incorrect diagnosis... So not only was my shoulder blade broken, my lowest disk also slipped out of the position and then broke after some time, the next two discs were protruding, in addition to having nerve channel inflammation and severe scoliosis. Seated meditation was no longer possible for me. Nevertheless, I told everyone that my spine would be better than ever within three years and that my scoliosis would be cured. Nobody believed me, as usual, and yet it came true.

Believe it or not, the accident saved my life, because I was with a Tibetan acupuncturist when the Tsunami in 2004 struck India; otherwise, I could have been one of the 250,000 victims.

In Thailand, I learned many techniques to improve life, health, and to gain more spirituality, from both Eastern and Western sources. I became a certificated life coach and EFT (Emotion Freedom Techniques) therapist. I fell in love with a beautiful, young Thai girl who was addicted to gambling. We struggled a lot to stop her addiction, and we are still together nine years later. Through her, I learned compassion and forgiveness. I earned my money on the stock market and have lived in Krabi, Thailand, for the last ten years.

I have coached a large number of people and have already prevented five suicides. I have recognized again and again the same mistakes that prevent people from living a happy life. Most people underestimate the influence of their subconscious minds, which control their whole lives. I have therefore written a book that teaches people how to live a happy and successful life, first in German, and then translated into English.

Never give up, and enjoy your life now. We never know what will happen next!

Table of Contents

Introduction

I was lying in a hospital in Krabi, Thailand, my entire body was paralyzed ... I could not believe that this had happened to me... I was 56 years old, and my body was fit and in top condition, able to compete in the mountains or swimming; in other words, my body was total healthy... and now this? I have been a raw food vegetarian (only fruits, vegetable, and nuts) for over 25 years, so a heart attack or stroke would be impossible because my blood is too thin for that...

The hospital staff was treating me like a piece of wood because I could not defend myself anymore. I thought about poor old people and how they get treated the same way... I had only one desire to go home... But how? To dead seem like it would be better and easier... when you can't feel anymore...

- During the entire time, I was repeating the name of God, so I remained relaxed.
- I have faith in God, so I was also thinking: thank you, God, that I was still alive.
- I had the desire to help people on their inner path, meaning that I still had a mission to live.

After some time I remembered the movie "The Secret", there was an episode with a guy who had an airplane crash, still alive, his body entirely paralyzed, nobody could help him; he had the single desire to leave the hospital, and 7 months later on Christmas... he did it!

How had this happened to me? That morning, I was using the toilet, and I saw that my eyes were swollen from the removal of the antifouling from the hulls of my catamaran... I felt quite bad, so I went back to bed, and then I experienced a fever attack, I could hardly make it to the bed. I was lying down, and then I decided that I needed help. So I phoned a friend of mine at 7 o'clock in the morning and asked her to please take me to the hospital... She said she had to take Oscar (her baby) to a friend's house first... in less than 10 minutes she was at my home with Oscar, and I could barely make it to her car, my body was so weak.

Fortunately, where is a will there is a way!

Then She was driving, and I got something like a stroke as I would touch 500 electric volts... I could not see anymore... she realized what was happening to me and went into panic mode... I could hear the screeching tires, the accelerating of the car, then came a second jolt/stroke, and my body became paralyzed.

 I asked where we were... she said to wait just a moment, then the third stroke hit, and my entire body was paralyzed...

The nightmare was just beginning, all the tests, including scanning of my brain, to assess the loss of oxygen to the brain, and the possible damage... I was in intensive care so they could not help me anymore. The staff was asking for money. They asked if I had enough money for the emergency ambulance ride to Phuket (2 ½ hours ride)

I wanted to go home and not to Phuket...my body was aching, I was laying on a hard plastic emergency bed...

I thought if the guy in "the secret" could do it, I as a highly spiritual being could too. I visualized leaving the hospital on my own feet... so I did 7 hours later... Still, I had to go to Phuket to be examined... they found out that it had been a cardiac arrest through cardiac arrhythmia which meant there was too less oxygen going to the brain... before that, I never was aware that I had a little heart rhythm problems.

 When I left the hospital, an old friend, Oskar, called me from Germany, he rarely called me (was it just a coincidence?)... I told him briefly what had happened, and he said: Again? I often made jokes about his hardships in life, because he had broken nearly every bone in his body, was a stunt man, a slaughter and a super agent (sabotage, espionage, killing) for the army. I understood I was not better than him, I had already been clinically dead 3 times, and faced death 4 times in the past 12 years... so what? He tried to make me laugh... yes I was quite traumatized.

Now we analyze this case.
1. I swim very fast every day for 30 to 40 minutes like a professional swimmer... it is hard to beat me!
2. I meditate every day for 2 hours.
3. I practice Chi Gong, stretching, and self massage every day for 1 hour.
4. I eat a raw food diet (only vegetable and fruits) for over 25 years, my body is in excellent condition!
5. My body is athletic, 192cm, and 74Kg.

After all of that, I found out later that I never can have a heart attack or stroke... So, then what happened to me?

Nearly every doctor would think that this case was impossible... Some days later, another friend asked me again and again what the reason for the cardiac arrest was. I was in a helpless situation 2 weeks ago, and that had caused the cardiac arrest.

There is a reason why we get a disease...

It is never a coincidence or some harmful viruses or bacteria that causes a disease! There are harmful viruses/bacteria everywhere in our environments, and everyday 13000 cancer cells attack our bodies, but not everybody is getting cancer!

Something is missing...

There is a way to help explain the phenomenon, psychosomatic, and scientific proofs that suppressed negative feelings are causing the diseases; Freud did research around this belief.

Suppressed negative feelings are causing the diseases

Stress is the number one killer

In this book, I will disclose many truths that western society and western medicine do not believe! Still, there is scientific proof about psychosomatic disorders. Please look it up on the Internet.

One honest word is more powerful than 1000 flattering words!

If you don't like to be offended with the truth, that is true, and has been for thousands of years:

In a healthy body, there is also a healthy spirit. -Hippocrates

In other words, most diseases are caused by suppressed negative feelings... I will prove that in this book!

I started my inner journey 30 years ago, with the German Book, "Krankheit als Weg"; the book was translated in English: "The Healing Power of Illness", it was a bestseller in Germany for 1 year. At that time, I was dealing with the challenges of a major health issue, and this book made it clear that 80% of all diseases are caused by suppressed negative feelings.
So I discovered and released my negative suppressed feelings, and I was even able to cure my epilepsy within half a year.

Today, I will take it one step further.

For example, ask yourself: What happens if…

1. I don't exercise?
2. I take drugs?
3. I live in a lousy environment?
4. I always eat junk food?
5. I smoke?
6. I work too many hours?
7. I bathe in the ocean in the winter time and catch a cold?

Why are you doing these and others that you know are not good for your health?

Because suppressed negative feelings are driving you to live this unhealthy life!

Consider this from another angle, there do exist people who are living an unhealthy lifestyle, but still, they are healthy. Germany was ruled by Chancellor Schmidt, he was born in 1918, he is still alive, and he is a chain smoker...or Mick Jagger (The Rolling Stones legend) born in 1943, is still performing on the stage and is well known for his drug excesses still he is alive...
There must be something more going on to explain what doesn't seem to make sense!

We need a reason to live and to enjoy our life

Once we have that, then we can overcome everything... and this is the reason why I am still alive, it is not my healthy lifestyle.

This book is about so much more too, I will show, for instance, how to cure your back and joint problems; a 100% cure for diabetes; show you that only a healthy lifestyle can heal your heart, and for cancer we need therapy. I will give you details about the best Chi Gong exercise from my book, Lean, to relax with meditation, and the best therapy to release your negative suppressed feelings with fast and easy steps with EFT from my book called: Enjoy your life now. For sure, there is also a chapter about the best food, and many links for getting your health back.

My mission is to make people happy and connect people to God.

I plan in the future to open a Holistic Health Center with Therapists, Tibetan, Ayurveda, Osteopathy, and Homeopathic Doctors...

Do you have an interest in learning more?

What is the cause and cure for diseases?

The causes of diseases are ignorance

(Ignorance means here, that we are not aware of our suppressed negative feelings) -Buddha

Before you cure the body, cure first the soul.

--Hippocrates

In a healthy body, there is also a healthy spirit.

--Esoteric

For Ayurveda, Chinese healing, Tibetan healing, Homeopathy, Bach flower therapy, and Osteopathy, the causes of diseases are suppressed negative feelings.

The causes of diseases are suppressed negative feelings, stress, unhealthy lifestyle, or sex-related.

--Mantak Chia and Osho

- Allergies – caused by totally suppressed anger.

- Asthma – caused by suppressed fear.
- Cancer – caused by all kinds of negative and suppressed feelings such as stress.
- Stomach, and Spleen problems like diabetes– caused by worry, grief, and taking life too seriously.
- Heart problems – caused by stress (stress is the outcome of suppressed fear and anger) or impatience (Thai: " yai ron" this means: "heart hot").
- Diarrhea – caused by fear and anxiety, as well as dodgy food.
- Lung problems – caused by depression.
- Kidney problems – caused by a deep fear or issues in a love relationship.
- Liver problems – caused by anger.

All of these diseases are also related to an unhealthy lifestyle.

See the end of the book for more about the diseases and the correlation of diseases.

The Cure

1. Look at which feelings or situations have caused the disease.
2. Release the suppressed negative feelings. Study the situation in-depth, relive it, and feel all the connected emotions. Or simply apply EFT (see more information at the end of this book) for every feeling in this/these situations.
3. If this is not working, go to a body and feelings orientated Therapist, like Bioenergetic, Biodynamic or EFT and tell him/her your problem
4. After the negative emotions are released, the body will heal by itself.

5. We can support the healing with Acupressure (read the book: "Acupuncture without needles"), Qigong, Reiki, Body exercise, Fresh Fruit and Vegetable juice, and massage
6. If we find out the cause of the disease and eliminate the reason, the body will heal. For instance:
shift work is extremely unhealthy, too less body exercise or junk food.

If we have pain:

If we have pain in an area of our body, we need to feel the pain with full awareness while looking for the specific place from which the pain originates. And then very often, the pain will go away by itself. This happens because we have accepted the pain. If we spend about 30 minutes intently focused on the source of the pain, that can be enough to make it vanish.

It is also true:

A chain is only as strong as its weakest link!

If we have a weak immune system, then we can potentially attract every possible disease.

Today are the reasons why so many people have a weak immune system:

1. the industrially processed food,
2. too little body exercise,
3. medications, drugs,
4. and stress.

If our immune system is weak, we are in a difficult or vulnerable situation:

1. one guy can get cancer,
2. another an allergy
3. or a heart attack.

I will go further with this concept, in the Chapter: The best Food, Prevention is Better than Medicine.
If we are ill, we should recognize and appreciate how our body has served us.

If our body is fit:

1. we are more relaxed,
2. vivid,
3. positive,
4. ore confident,
5. and we have more power to accomplish our goals.

If we are ill we ask ourselves:

1. Why do we exploit our body?
2. Do we exploit our body for meaningless reasons?
3. Are we looking for substitutes for happiness, when we mistreat our body?
4. Why can't we make daily exercise part of our regular routine?
5. Why can't we stick to a healthy diet?
6. Do we want to suffer because of the food we eat and our lack of exercise?

In the ancient world when the Greeks were ruling the western world, there was an emperor who wanted to get rid of his camp of foreigners. What did he do? To kill them would be too harsh, so he said to them, within a half year you will die. I don't want to kill you right now, so I have decided that within a half year you will get on one day poisoned food. In the meantime, you should enjoy your life. After one week all the foreigners were dead, even without getting any poison. How weird the emperor thought, maybe somebody had poisoned them without his permission. So he tried it again on another group of foreigners. This time he required a member of his staff to eat the same food as the people in the group of foreigners. The result was the same, the foreigners died within one week, but not his staff member. He made even stricter rules for the next groups, and the results remained the same. Then he understood that:

Fear is the best poison to kill people

In the USA they found, that if a patient had incurable cancer, but did not know about it, they would die much later than the patients who knew they were sick. Even many patients didn't die!

If this is true, with faith, we can cure diseases. Every disease that has a cure or even those without treatment can be healed through faith.

Faith is the best remedy for all diseases, without faith, no disease can be cured.

The most important thing is that the doctor or healer gives the patient hope and faith.

The next problem is that if a person has no mission or a particular reason or fun to live for, then a severe disease can kill him. This might be the reason why many people just die when they are diagnosed with a challenging illness. They don't choose the best treatment, even if it is working. To persuade them to change the treatment is very difficult because they want to die. If we see this, then the psychological reason for choosing the right treatment is essential! Otherwise, we will die.

For many chronic diseases, there is no cure because the patients want to keep this disease in order:

1. To get compassion/love from their family and friends.
2. To have a reason not to work.
3. To press his/her environment for doing something for him/her.
4. To be important.
5. The next reason is that the patient is overloaded with problems so that they can't follow a diet, medical cure, or they are not open for alternative healing, then it is easier to take pills.

There is a cure for every disease

The problem is who has enough power to do so?
Do we have enough reason or a mission to live to do so?

What is Phantom Pain?

Phantom pain is a pain that is continuous, even after the treatment when there is no reason for the pain anymore. For instance, if we have a particle in our eyes and we remove it, but still there is a pain. The same is valid for back pain and many other diseases. Even after many years, we can have phantom pain, for an already cured disease. The pain is something individual and connected with the psychology of the patient.

I had known quite a lot of medical students, that when they studied the different diseases, they directly examined their own body. And thought that they had each disease that they learned about during the previous lesson. They even got the symptoms.

Or we had a horse, and we wanted her to get pregnant, so she was implanted with the semen and got all symptoms of pregnancy, but she never got pregnant.
This is pure psychology, we imagine something, and then it seems to materialize or come into being.

What is a placebo?

In the '70s there was a scandal about a doctor who took huge fees to cure impotence in London/ England. He cured 60% of the impotence of males that nobody else could heal. What was the problem? The other 40% still paid the doctor's fee and didn't get cured. They went to court and complained about this doctor. The doctor asked what more could they want, he said that he had cured 60% of his clients and that it is an excellent result. The judge said: you only gave patients an injection of water and dextrose for huge fees! The doctor said the treatment doesn't matter because I have cured them!

From this time on, western doctors saw every medical treatment that worked and was not 100% scientifically proven as a placebo effect!

Today it is proven by science that the placebo effect is a good cure because we don't need any medications, and still, it works for 20% to 60% of the cases, depending on the diagnose and the patient.

Wow, the expectation of getting healed is more important than the actual medical treatment!!!!!!!!!!

In the old Chinese times, there was this great yellow emperor. China was running out of medications for malaria when malaria got worse. The yellow emperor recommended simply that we don't need this medication; just repeat again and again the name of the medication and imagine that you are taking the drug. And his idea worked. I have tried this, too; instead of taking antibiotics for an infection, and this worked for me.

26

If we think it over for several diseases, it is crucial that the doctor convinces the patient that his treatment is working.

For instance, the doctor says the chance that you will survive is X% when you take his treatment; without treatment, you will die.

The patient gets even more anxious… Why did the doctor say anything about the chance to survive?

The ultimate health formula

Ask yourself if you want to cure your disease:

1. What disease would you like to cure?

2. What are the possible reasons that you got this disease; for instance, stress, shift work, unhealthy lifestyle or you don't like your job or work environment? For 2 minutes, think and feel about the reason/reasons and write them down.

3. What is the cause of this disease? Which feelings did you suppress so that you got this disease? Think and feel about it and write it down.

4. Is this disease related to some other illness or circumstances? If yes, then also look at the other diseases.

5. Most people who have a chronic disease don't want to get it cured. Think about what benefit you gain or have for keeping this disease. For instance, people caring for you; a reason why you don't have to work?

6. What disadvantages do you have from this disease? Make a list.

7. Imagine you will be ill for the rest of your life and suffering from this disease, perhaps you will die soon because the disease is getting worse, feel it and write it down.

8. Imagine that you get cured and can live a happy life so that you can create every moment new, you can enjoy the here and now;

you will choose your perfect job, environment, a healthy lifestyle, and will have a great loving relationship. Feel it.

9. You release the suppressed feelings. You decide to change your life to become healthy. And this is the cure.

10. You have faith that you can cure it, and think about the people who have already done so. You accept the disease with all its symptoms. If not, make a fear list and do EFT for every fear. Without faith, it is hardly possible to cure any severe disease.

11. You support the healing with alternative healing that has fewer side effects like body exercise, fresh juices, raw foods, Reiki, Chinese healing with acupressure, and Qigong.

12. You eliminate the cause of that illness, for instance: relationship problems, stress, shift work, and unhealthy environments.

My strategy to convince everybody that their disease can be cured:

A friend had to undergo heart surgery with the chance of survival only 20%. I told him that he needed a reason to live for, and to think over what he wanted to do after recovering from the surgery. After 14 days in a coma, he regained consciousness and changed his entire life.

Stress is the killer number one!

Is really our stress necessary?

So more stress we have, so more we fail, so more our body is suffering, so more our relationships are getting worse… and we attract so more bad things/dramas in our life….

How to get rid of it. We start first with our own lives, what we can improve… If we have not enough fun or playtime, then we procrastinate, and with procrastination, we are getting the stress…. First, we schedule our free time… because free time is more than anything else important. If we can't enjoy our free time or have not enough free time, then we procrastinate and then the stress….

We chose after the 20% to 80% rule… (that 20% of the doing brings 80% of the success) what is the most important things to do and we do it right away?
Before we are starting to work, we think Why or what is the reason to do our task… Because if we don't have a strong Why, then we are not motivated to do the job… Do we need really to make everything or is 20% just enough?

After every task, we take a pause and think how good it was that we have done it… It is okay if we can do some relaxing exercises, like breathing, a short walk after the task,… Because it will clear our mind from unnecessary thoughts. We choose not to work overtime because then we have to less free time…

After and before our work, body exercise will help us a lot to be relaxed.
I had always chosen to go by bicycle to my job…. Then we can look at what kind of relationship we need and what type of relationship will exhaust us…

This means we should get rid of stress-makers… We want a happy life, for this, we should also choose the right people and to be together out of politeness with the wrong people, doesn't make sense.

To learn to meditate also makes sense. If we start with meditation, then we should begin with moving meditation, like the Kundalini Mediation from Osho.

The western medicine kills us

783,936 people in the United States die every year from conventional medicine mistakes.

According to the groundbreaking 2003 medical report, Death by Medicine, by Drs. Gary Null, Carolyn Dean, Martin Feldman, Debora Rasio, and Dorothy Smith, 783,936 people in the United States die every year from conventional medicine mistakes. That's the equivalent of six jumbo jet crashes a day for an entire year. But where is the media attention for this tragedy? Where is the government support for stopping these medical mistakes before they happen?

Learn more:
http://www.naturalnews.com/009278.html#ixzz3KcnmGYMx

   http://www.collective-evolution.com/2013/05/07/death-by-prescription-drugs-is-a-growing-problem/

Out of the 783,936 annual deaths from conventional medicine mistakes, approximately 106,000 of those are the result of prescription drug use [1]. According to the Journal of the American Medical Association, two-hundred, and ninety people in the United States are killed by prescription drugs every day [4].
In the EU, over 200000 (50000 in Germany) people are dying every year from the side effects of medications.
In Germany every year, there are 15000 people killed through doctor's mistakes. It is a fact that German doctors are killing more people than any terrorist organization! And 12500 more people die from particular viruses in hospitals (44 people every day) in Germany. And these numbers are the official numbers, the real numbers are 2 or 3 times higher!

Western medicine doesn't view the body, soul, and mind as one unit

Western medicine views the body like a butcher who sees the meat and not the suffering of the animals. Western medicine disregards the pain of the soul and mind.

Western medicine does not look for the cause of diseases. They treat symptoms without knowing the cause of the diseases. This never can be a science, it is pseudo science.

It is rather more an empirical science and not a logical science. I will prove this in the chapter about the Heart. Through trial and error, they try to heal the patients. What was true 20 years ago is often wrong today. For instance, all medications for heart harm more often than they improve the heart. Dr. John Bergman proves this in his Youtube channel after the new scientific results.

Western medicine is fighting against the symptoms instead of healing them!

The cure is really that the:

- Symptoms are suppressed through the treatments with the side effect of a weaker immune system. In the end, these treatments will kill the patients! (Dr. John Bergman).
- Or that the symptoms from an unhealthy organ will be shifted to the healthy organs so that in the end, nothing is accomplished. Also, the immune system continues to get weaker.

Western medicine always makes our immune system weaker and slows our metabolic rate.

See metabolism Wikipedia.
The building up of new cells called anabolism and the breaking down of cells called catabolism. For the building up of new cells, we need the enzymes as a catalyst. We are healthy if we have a reasonable metabolism/ metabolic rate, then we build up more cells than breaking down of cells. See: Chapter Prevention is better than medicine; - What makes our immune system strong?

When I was traveling with Amma (Mata Amritananda Mai) through India, 20 years ago; we had to make malaria prophylaxis for Bombay. When I looked up the side effects of the prophylaxis, I was shocked. I realized that getting malaria would be better than to take the prophylaxis, even though all western doctors strongly recommend taking it. I never took the malaria prophylaxis when I was traveling several times a year to Bombay, and I never got malaria even with so many mosquitoes in Bombay. It was not the case with the people who took the malaria prophylaxis, 5% got malaria. In other words, the prophylaxis just means big money for the pharmaceutical industry!

Western Doctors

The typical western doctor's practice is set up so that every doctor has 2 to 3 waiting rooms for treatment and then the doctors jump from one room to the next room to serve as many patients as possible. Also, their staff members have one of the lowest salaries in Germany.
If we see how time and money are optimized in the clinics, I question their motivation for working as doctors; do they really like helping people, or is money much more vital to them.

Do you think that medical Doctors want to help patients with chronic diseases or severe diseases? From them, they can make big money with less effort. I would like to come back to the placebo effect, do you think that Doctors try to persuade the patients that their treatment is working? Never, because then they would lose their income and also their time would not be as valuable!!!!! And for them, time is **Money Money Money.**

If we take more than 3 different medications daily, then the risk for dementia is considerable.

Here are the annual numbers from the USA according to health insurance companies

1. Dementia is the highest annual bill for health insurance companies in the USA.
2. 28% of hospitalizations among seniors are due to adverse drug reactions.
3. 65 to 69 years old are taking over 14 prescriptions a year.
4. 80 to 84 years old are taking more than 18 prescriptions per year.
5. 1 of 3 Americans has heart disease, cancer, high blood pressure, or diabetes.
6. 1 of 4 Americans has a mental health disorder in the USA.
7. 2007 50% of US children have a chronic disease/disorder because of vaccines and genetically modified food.
8. 2013 21% of US children have Autism, ADHD, or another developmental disability.
9. By 2016 60% to 70% of US children are chronically ill, obesity, and infertility.

10. After new research, children without taking vaccines are simple healthy… see Youtube John Bergman https://www.youtube.com/watch?v=BQeA9ZzSAXo

11. After research, if we inject two different viruses as a vaccine/s in the blood within several weeks, then the immune system can't cope that, and severe diseases can happen. A newborn baby is getting within 18 months 12 vaccines….

Western medicine makes us ill!

We are now in the darkest time of Western medicine, where the doctors, the medicaments, the industrially processed food, genetically modified food causing most of the severe diseases.

The reason is simple, so more patience, so more money is making the doctors and the pharmaceutic industry. Our politicians know this already, and they even support this with new laws for making more money for the doctors and pharmaceutic industry.

- President Obama supported the vaccination, health (hells) care… and junk food like Hod Dogs for students…. If we don't protest against these (doctors, medicaments, the industrially processed food, genetically modified food), then the next generation will suffer a lot from that!!!!

Read more about that in the Cancer chapter.

The Tibetan medicine

Tibetan medicine heals sixty percent of the chronic diseases that are not curable by Western medicine (TV report in Germany). Therefore, Tibetan healing is the most successful healing! Tibetan healing is used to balance the different energies in the body and the organs, it cures with acupuncture or herbs, like Chinese healing. They are using alternative therapies like acupuncture and herbs (they are using different herbs than the Chinese).

When I have gone to Tibetan doctors, they give patients the confidence that they can cure your diseases. And they do. They have time for you and answer your questions. The methods I prefer are acupuncture or cupping because they do not have side effects. For my back, they have done an excellent job. The best Tibetan doctors live in Dharamsala, where the Dalai Lama lives.

I was also in Lhasa/Tibet. Here the Tibetan doctors are under the control of the Chinese government, and they can't practice their own style.
The Tibetan doctors like to give intuitive Acupuncture based on feeling the patient's pulse, but that is not allowed in China; only acupuncture based on the official charts for every disease is recommended.

The Indian Ayurveda

Ayurveda is so complex that it is hard to understand for me.

I often went to an ancient Ayurveda Doctor who was one of the best in India.

When I entered the room, he already knew what problem I had. One time when I entered the room, he said I had hemorrhoids. He was really amazing. The medications worked well but tasted really awful.

Even for a very bad wound infection, the herbs work.

Nevertheless, most of the Ayurveda medications have awful side effects.

If you want to start with Ayurveda, You should make first a whole-body purification with the Panchakarma treatment.

The Panchakarma treatment also includes massage and all organ cleanings, and you need for this treatment 4 weeks.

And the Panchakarma treatment heals very many diseases…

In South India, Kerala is suitable for Ayurveda treatments… The Ashram of Mata Amritanandamayi (Kerala/Kollam/Parayakadavu) offers one of the best Panchakarma treatment and one of the best Ayurveda doctor).

The very best Ayurveda doctor Triguna died with over 100. And now, his sons are treating the patients well.

Vaid Brihaspati DevTriguna Clinic Sarai Kale Khan
4.5(88) · Alternative medicine practitioner

New Dehli/ close to Railwaystation Nizamuddin
19-A, Railway Crossing, Sarai Kale Khan, Near, Nizamuddin E Ln
+91 11 2435 1221

https://www.google.co.th/maps/dir/8.1477524,98.8867707/ayurvedic
+doctor+triguna+in+delhi/@28.5835199,77.2528863,17.32z/data=!4
m9!4m8!1m1!4e1!1m5!1m1!1s0x390ce30c1fa98e8d:0x51666a67a33
47685!2m2!1d77.2552303!2d28.584545

Prevention is better than medicine

Historically in China, the healer kept the people healthy; if they got diseases, he was replaced.

A pleasant environment is a must for good health!

If we are living in situations with conflicts that we hardly can bear, then we will eventually get diseases and get sick from that environment.

A conflict that we can't bear will make us ill!

What should we do if we are in a lousy conflict or stressful situation?

1. We need to solve this conflict.
2. We can get away from this conflict, through maybe changing the environment, or ending bad relationships.
3. We let go of this conflict! When we are doing body and feelings orientated therapy, like EFT (described in this book), we can easily let go of this conflict. The best solution is to go to see a therapist.

Most of the things that we chase are not worth the stress.

If we think about all the bad situations that we have faced over the years, we can really evaluate whether these conflicts were worth all the stress, desperation, anger, and sadness. Most of the time, we will discover that they were not worth our anguish. Is it not wiser to leave the situation sooner rather than later, even if we are losing face?

You can be right or happy

All these disputes are unnecessary most of the time, it is far better to just leave the situation and move on.

 When I was fifteen years old, I made my apprenticeship as a telecommunication installer far away from home. The masters in this firm were cruel and tried their best to make lives horrible for the apprentices. I could not bear their unjust and unfair behavior. It drove me nearly to suicide.

Then I learned autogenous training and positive thinking. With positive thinking, I brought my mind and feelings under my control. And later, I was diagnosed with epilepsy.

If we apply positive thinking for suppressing our negativity, we will get severe diseases!
Positive thinking is only suitable for giving our life a focus.

In the last discussion I had about this with Brendon Burchard, he still thinks positive thinking is working, even though he had a brain tumor! I fore-casted that every great positive thinker would get cancer because of suppressing his negative feelings.
Until now, with this quote, I am right.

The most reputable firm for seminars is Success Resources, which was started by the billionaire, Richard Tan, who I know personally also had cancer.

After the apprenticeship, I liked to study. First, I had to go back to school, and then as an a student, I studied Electrotechnique. Again, I got into big arguments with my teachers because of their unjust and unfair behavior. I went to the student Parliament and won my case. After that, all the teachers disliked me.

Nevertheless, I founded a new party and won the majority in the student parliament election. Although that sounds good, I nearly died through this experience, because of too much stress. My face was paralyzed. And from an incorrect medical treatment, I became clinical dead, and left my body and came back after some time.

And then I made this decision:

My life should be the sum of my happiness!

Nothing is more important than to be happy in the here and now!

We chase things in our lives, and we can't even remember why!

What is better, a ton of money and a life full of stress; or to be relaxed, happy, healthy, and to have a loving relationship?

After this study, I began to study psychology on my own. Still, I had many diseases, and I wanted to cure them. I read this excellent book, "Krankheit als Weg". (Engl. Translation: "The Healing Power of Illness" still, you can buy it in English.). This book explains that nearly 80% of the diseases are psychosomatic (caused by suppressed negative feelings).

I participated in 'body and feelings' orientated therapy groups, Qigong, and meditation. And with this approach I cured my body.

We can cure our diseases with 'body and feelings' orientated therapy!

How can we boost our immune system?

It is not difficult to understand why managers and even every president of the USA jogs, it is because it makes the body much stronger. We can also get rid of our stress and aggression through running, and if we do it even when it is raining, snowing, and cold, then we will get a strong body!

Jogging and riding a bicycle daily in any weather or skillful swimming makes everybody strong!

Then I started going on extended meditation retreats first in Germany and then in India. During this time, I became a raw food eater (only fruits, vegetables, and nuts). Since then, I have stayed on the plan of the Natural Hygiene Society (NHS) their society has been around for 200 years, and people who follow their recommendations live 25 years longer than the average.

In addition, everybody should have enough sunlight, time to rest, and regular exercise for their body. Then all the diseases will disappear.

I had the optimal lifestyle, but still, I frequently caught colds and other minor diseases.

I found out that my optimal lifestyle would boost my body but could not prevent diseases!

An optimal lifestyle with the best food and exercise can't prevent diseases!

In India, it was too hot for jogging, so I swam every day, did my bioenergetic work, as well as Qigong, and Thai Chi. Through sitting for long periods, I got pain in my legs. I learned Acupressure from the book: "Acupuncture without needles". I learned to give myself a full body massage when necessary.

When our Ashram was on the tour of North India in the wintertime, nearly 66% of the people caught a cold including me, because we were living in the warm mild climate of Kerala. In the meantime, I had learned Acupressure quite well and applied it the next time I noticed the beginning of symptoms for a cold. As a result, I didn't get sick. Acupressure works for many diseases.

Acupressure or a good self-massage from Mantak Chia can boost our body's energy tremendously!

Later, I had an accident, and a disk in my lower back was broken. With the Chinese healing of Acupuncture, Acupressure, Self-massage, and Qigong from Mantak Chia, I cured my back.

I learned the inner organ massage, Tao love, Microcosmos, 5 Elements, Iron shirt III, and the previous Iron shirt II from Mantak Chia, all are awesome.

How to live longer through longevity genes?

Put your body through pain throughout your live that will activate your genes for longevity… (Dr. David Sinclair Harvard, Professor of genetics)

Today they can grow in the lab a brain; age it and increase the longevity.
Even a blind rat could grow back its factuality to see again…

And this they have done with the 7 longevity genes…

All great stuff…

The idea to live longer means that we stay younger for a longer period of time without suffering through diseases… and then we should die fast in a healthy matter.
Today is it rather so that we suffer for many years through diseases and that we keep us alive by medicaments… And that is wrong!

Dr. Sinclair recommendations:

What don't kill you, makes you live longer.

This means controlled pain, for instance: just go in the sauna afterward in an ice-bath and then make your workouts…

What makes the body strong helps for longevity and activates the longevity genes.

Make Highly intensive training… lose your breath once go over your limit…
Or you make this high cold training, you stay in a cold place/water for some time… like the "Wim Hof' method" this is all science proved for many decades.

The idea is, you should go into survival mode.
Then your longevity genes kicks in.

Convenience, comfortableness makes your body weak…

Stay hungry without getting malnutrition…
Instead of eating, you fill your stomach with warm water/green tea/juice.
If we skip a meal or fast our longevity genes gets activated…
That is all true!

For instance, they have done surveys with mice, dogs and monkeys…
One group stayed comfortable and convenience with food.
And the other group stayed hungry…
Guess which group has done it better… 20% longer life…

I disagree with his other food recommendation, because they are his private recommendation and they are not based on science…!

He recommends High carbon food or High fat food (pure olive oil) - but that needs a long digest time and that is in any case bad, and doesn't make sense for skipping one meal.
We should fill up our stomach only up to 60% and with 1 meal daily, we cannot survive with a low carbon and low-fat diet…

The trueness is, the raw coast eater, fruit vegetarians have the longest life span, 25 years longer life span than average people…. And that is still the best! For sure they don't eat grains or fatty food, only a handful of nuts is allowed… and even this I don't do!

His next recommendations are:
No smoking.
Vegetarian food.
Organically grown food.
Colored vegetables/fruits.
Green leafy vegetables.

Get a good night's sleep…
Surround yourself with good people, friends that care for you…
Yes, that is all good…

The best remedies to drink…

Best in the morning for boosting up the immune system…

Make ginger/ lemon juice at least 3/4l.

Heat water up to 50 Celsius not higher!
Grind ginger and put so much ginger inside so that it doesn't get too spicy.
Wait 10 minutes.
Add lemon juice so it doesn't get too acid…
Filter/sieve out the ground ginger
And ad honey…

If you cached a cold/ virus infection…

Heat water up to 50 Celsius not higher, at least 1/2l!
Grind ginger and put so much ginger inside so that it doesn't get too spicy…
Put Thyme so much inside that it will still taste good…
Wait 10 minutes.
Add lemon juice so it doesn't get too acid…
Ad honey…

Thyme is the very best herb for respiratory diseases/virus infection, ginger will kill all bacteria…
And then drink it on an empty stomach.

Kidney/bladder:

Get 100 to 150 gr. Dried Cranberry…
Cover them with warm water, up to 50 Celsius…100 to 150ml water.
(Never cook any fruits, it is the worst for the Kidneys, besides
Coffee!)
Ad Apple (cider) vinegar 10 to 15ml….
Wait 10 minutes…
Blend it until it is smooth and looks delicious like a baby pudding!
Add 200 - 300ml water… If you fill before the first blending the 200
to 300ml water, you never get it smooth like a baby pudding.
Blend it again.

Make ginger/ lemon juice at least 1/2l
Heat water up to 50 Celsius not higher!
Grind ginger and put so much ginger inside so that it doesn't get too
spicy.
Wait 10 minutes
Add lemon juice so it doesn't get too acid…
Filter/sieve out the ground ginger
And ad honey…

And then drink both on an empty stomach…

Inactivity is a major cause of death…

Insights (TED) of a 93-year-old man who makes bodybuilding …

When we had been hunters to find food, we had only a chance to survive when we tried our best physically and mentally … After we killed that animal, we had to eat as much as possible to sustain our body as long as possible; and to relax to be inactive to gain our power back…

So what, overeating was a must …
Inactivity was a must to relax…

And these necessary habits are destroying us today.

And today we overeat and be inactive even we didn't do any exercise…

Successful aging is possible:

Three factors are contributing to successful aging and guess that are using the Japanese with the highest longevity… (50000 Japanese are over 100 years old)

1. work hard
2. right diet
3. body exercise

The aged person is suffering from inactivity, poor diet, overweight, diabetes …And this happened through retirement.

Retirement is voluntary or involuntary unemployment for up to 30 years…

Unemployment cause:

1. Chronic disease
2. Mental problems
3. Poor health
4. Disabilities
5. More medical consultation
6. More hospital admissions

For what is work good?

1. Work is therapeutic
2. Good for health
3. Self-worth
4. Family esteem
5. Identity
6. Standing in the community

Inactivity kills

The aged people should be integrated into the workforce for health reasons as it was 100 years ago.

Exercise is both a preventive measure and treatment.

The motivation can be:
to be sexier
or vanity.

People who exercise in strenuous competitive sports live longer.

With 80 years the body has lost 50% of the muscle strength of a 50 years-old-person…
Just train and get your muscles back…

You can rebuild your body at any age…

Get your Sleep

Doctors who are addicted to work, say we need only 6 hours of sleep. But typically doctors say we need 8 hours. So, it depends on the person. It is essential to get the right amount of sleep; to go to bed between 10pm and 11pm. Otherwise, we don't get our so necessary REM sleep cycle. A nap during daytime hours is also good. Sleeping pills are working against us because we don't get our REM sleep cycle.

What Makes Our Immune System Weak?

1. Stress
2. Depression
3. Anger
4. Too little exercise
5. Too much sex
6. Time spent with bad people
7. An unhealthy environment where you work and live
8. Western medicine
9. Drugs including smoking and coffee
10. Industrially processed food, because it is dead food without enzymes
11. Pizza with cheese, over-baked food, twice or more heated up food
12. White sugar
13. Pies, Tarts, Cookies, Cakes, junk food
14. Shift work

To 5. Too much sex drains the body and weakens the body. Everybody has to find out for themselves what is too much or too less sex.

To 6. Wicked people will pull us down emotionally and negatively affect our immune system.

To 7. It is proven that when we work in a beautiful, healthy place, then we are much more motivated than if we work in a dirty, loud, and unhealthy area. It also affects our immune system. Offices that offer employees a pleasant, healthy environment to work reduced the diseases by 50 %.

And with Feng Shui, it is getting even much better! Feng Shui creates a beautiful and cozy atmosphere that supports our health, success…

To 8. Western medicine is like shooting at a bird with a nuclear bomb. It destroys our good well organized immune system. For an instant, with the antibiotics, we kill our healthy bacteria, so that the harmful bacteria will grow in our guts. Actually, we need the bacteria in our body, only some bacteria are harmful.

You will find the following points in the food chapter.

What makes our immune system strong?

1. Love
2. Happiness
3. Enough sex
4. Massage
5. Enough exercise
6. Qigong and Yoga
7. Meditation and prayer
8. Good healthy environment
9. Enough rest
10. Enough sunlight
11. Fresh sprouts
12. Fresh pressed juice from vegetable and fruits
13. Raw foods
14. Vegetables cooked with grains or potatoes
15. Superfoods like raw unprocessed cacao powder, wheatgrass, and spirulina powder…

Everything you want to know about food...

The best Food

In the media, we read so much contrary information about the best diet, and it's very confusing.

First, consider who is writing about the healthy diet and what the author wants to promote and how much commission he is getting. That makes at least ninety percent of the articles written about diet useless.

Meat-eating is not suitable for our body
Our teeth are not designed for eating raw meat.

Have you eaten raw meat that is not cut into small pieces? A meat-eater, like a lion, only has 5 meter-long bowels (humans have 12 meter-long guts, which are the best for vegetables and fruits) and all meat eaters have stronger and better-suited teeth, as well as a bigger mouth in relation to their body. Our teeth are suitable for eating vegetables, fruits, and nuts.

We also have problems eating uncooked grains with our teeth, like wheat and rice. Naturally, we are vegetable, fruit, seed, and nut eaters.

A vegetarian lives on average five to ten years longer

(see Wikipedia Vegetarianism).

See: http://michaelbluejay.com/veg/natural.html

A vegetarian will have a major digestive problem if he or she eats meat after not eating it for five years; it can cause food poisoning.

Eating meat is not natural for us. In the meat/seafood that we get in the supermarket is antibiotics, in order to keep the animals healthy; synthetic estrogen and other hormones to grow them faster; dioxins; pesticides; inorganic arsenic (in chicken, that can cause cancer, dementia, …) heavy metals and very many other toxic from unhealthy food given to the animals. See for instance: http://www.peta.org/living/food/meat-contamination/ ; http://www.zentrum-der-gesundheit.de/muell-als-viehfutter-ia.html .

The antibiotics (read next chapter) in the meat that we eat, kill the good bacteria in our intestines so that our immune system is getting weak. Not all the bacteria can be destroyed from the antibiotics.-

Harmful and dangerous bacteria developed through antibiotics in the industrially processed food and meat/fish. Now we have bacteria that are resistant to antibiotics and even bacteria (Superbug) that can kill us, and we have no remedy against them. These Superbugs are inside of the eggs, meat, fish, shrimps, and milk. Please avoid shrimps, crabs, lobster, shellfish because of the bad bugs!

In addition for one-kilo meat, we need 6000Gal water (the USA will lacking on groundwater in 10 to 20 years because of the cows and pigs) and up to 20kg food….

What do they feed our cattle/farmed fish, poultry?
The pig's food can be glycerin, sludge, meat and fish waste.
The cattle's food can be chicken shit, slop from bio-diesel, meat waste, genetically modified corn (quite toxic);
And for the farmed shrimps/fish are the antibiotics and fish waste.

If we see how the animals are treated from producers for meat/eggs/milk, then it is a no-brainer to stop eating meat.
Or just visit a chicken or a pig farm and see what happens there or go to a slaughter. **Bone appetite**.

The producers of meat/eggs/milk pollute our rivers/groundwater/farmland with their feces.

The US-farmers must accept, that the producer of meat/eggs/milk can put the toxic wastes on their ground and the toxic will be later in our vegan food.

There is a real story, a chicken farmer put his feces in the Dümmer See (North Germany) and afterward, was the sea with a surface of $13.5Km^2$ biological dead for 10 years ….

Imagine, that the cows eating feces.
How much the producers of eggs pollute our water and land?

A raw food eater lives twenty to thirty years longer

A raw food eater lives twenty to thirty years longer (see https://www.healthscience.org) on average. Why? For instance, if we give a duck bread, then its lifespan is reduced by fifty percent. The reason is that a duck cannot digest the salt and cooked grains in the bread, and all the vitamins and nutrition are destroyed in the bread through processing. In Germany, it is forbidden to give ducks bread. With raw food, we have much more energy and also much more emotions and feelings; it is easier to meditate. If we eat fruits and salad, then our digestion happens very fast, the process typically takes only thirty minutes, whereas typical cooked food takes 4 to 24 hours to digest.

The body of a raw food eater is basic

The body produces acidic gastric juices for meat, cooked food, and alkaline gastric juices for all raw food, except raw meat and different nuts, seeds, beans. If we have eaten mainly food that needs acid gastric juices our body is acidic and vice versa for alkaline gastric juices.

If we make a urine test and pie on a litmus paper, then we see how basic or acidic is our body. For a meat-eater is the pH 4-5, for a raw food eater pH 7-9. Meat-eaters have a very acidic body, they attract quite a lot of diseases like: joins problems, because of the acidic crystal's in their joints; kidney problems, heart attack, brain stroke, cancer, diabetes, dementia from their acidic and thick blood.

We need seventy percent of our energy to digest typical cooked meals, then for sure, there is not much energy left for our emotions. The raw food eater needs only 10% of his energy for the digestion and has so much more power for his life and feelings.

The majority of people like to eat when they want to suppress their negative feelings (anger, sadness, and fear); which explains why so many people are fat.

Our habit is to eat cooked food. Adhering to a raw-food diet is considered too difficult, and no one would believe that it could make us happy. Our society would not accept it, and people who tried it would feel isolated. I know this from experience since I have been a raw-food eater for 30 years.

Metabolism

The metabolism of our body breakdowns our food and transform it into energy. The building up of new cells is called anabolism, and the breaking down of cells is also called catabolism.
For the building up of new cells, we need the enzymes as a catalyst.

So more enzymes we have in our food so faster we build up new cells.

All fresh raw food has enough enzymes, cooked food has no enzymes.
If we have a good metabolism/metabolic rate; then we build up more cells than breaking down of cells.
If we are healthy, then we produce more cells than cells are dying.
See:
Chapter: *Prevention is better than medicine*; - *What makes our immune system strong?*

Genetically modified food

The European Union made 19 studies in 2011, for feeding genetically modified soybean and maize to mammals. After 6 months, 43% of the males had kidney diseases and 30.8% of the female's liver diseases. The USA is the biggest Corn producer of the world and had delivered their genetically modified (GM) corn to China. China rejected this GM Corn, so did Russia and Japan, 2013. There must be a reason for this! If an insect is eating this corn, it will die from the toxic inside of the corn.

After medical research, when a pregnant woman is eating meat from GM Corn fed cow, the later newborn baby will have the toxic inside of his blood….

What should we eat?

1.   If we want to be kind to our body, then a detox treatment with fruits and exercise for our body is good.

2.   Eat fruits before the main meal, and not together with cooked food; otherwise, the fruit will ferment. Wait until the fruit is digested and then you can eat cooked food.

3.   Avoid white sugar (white poison).

4.   The industrial processed oils and fats that are used mostly everywhere, be it in the salad dressing or as margarine or the cooking oil for the meat... is very bad... like poison. It can clog our arteries in our heart. For instance, the so-called salad oil: the producers use paint thinner to get the last drop of the oil out of seeds. Instead of them use only cold-pressed oil, fish oil or butter.

5.   Avoid oily and greasy foods, both will make digestion so difficult. For example, just one tablespoon of oil makes digestion take two hours longer! And it will also make you put on weight.

6.   Avoid all cooked fruits, including tomatoes, cucumbers, and capsicum because they are then very acidic for the body.

7.   Avoid meat because it harms the heart, and makes the body acidic.The biggest problem in becoming a vegetarian is that most people are unable to cook vegetarian food. Vegetarian food is very delicious, nearly everyone who tries it likes it, and I could easily convince you with my cooking (I enjoy cooking for other people). It's simple to learn how to cook vegetarian food.

8.   Avoid heavy food like pizza (requires twenty-four-hours to be digested), tarts, cheese over baked food, French fries, mayonnaise, too many spices, chilies and coffee.

9.   If we want to live even healthier, then have fruits for breakfast and no coffee. Before breakfast, exercise your body and meditate so that your body can detox every morning. The fiber of the fruits will clean our arteries.

10.   Drink a lot of pure water daily, 2 liters/day is perfect. In the morning start with two glasses of warm water.

11.   There is this outdated and incorrect belief that we need a lot of protein. A baby needs much more protein than a grown-up. And breast milk has only 1.5% protein. Most fruits, vegetables, or nuts have more protein than 1.5%, even tomatoes have 3% fully adequate protein, bananas have up to 10%. In the history of medicine, there was not a person who got sick from too little protein. Actually, if you give the chicken a lot of protein, they produce more eggs. It is similar for human beings, an overdose of protein, meaning more than10g of protein will create more lust because the males will produce more semen and the female more moisture in their vagina.

12.   Industrially manufactured food is typically unhealthy and acidic. First, you don't know how the food has been processed. For instance, they found eggshells in the best brand of noodles from Germany. Then they found out they use the broken eggs from the farmers, including all the dirt to manufacture their noodles. Plus, there is no energy in the food. Also, there are no enzymes in this food. **We need enzymes for our digestion and for our immune system. Vitamins are not enough for a healthy body, without the enzymes we can't absorb the vitamins in our body!** If it is written with added vitamins, without the enzymes we can't absorb the vitamins. If there would be enzymes in the industrially processed food, then the food will be perishable. That means that the Industrially

manufactured food will weaken our immune system and destroy the healthy balance of good and not so beneficial bacteria in our bowels.

13.   Dairy products are produced from heated and processed milk so that all the benefits are gone, instead of giving the body calcium. The processed milk is draining calcium out of the body; the cheese is processed with antibiotics or they even use radioactivity to keep it fresh longer. The curd/sour cream is still beneficial because it gives us calcium.

14.   The healthiest foods are sprouts and wheatgrass. In 100 grams, there is enough to cover all our vitamin needs for the day and almost enough protein too. We can grow sprouts ourselves, and they are very cheap. We just need to buy the seeds and put them in water.

15.   Fresh juice out of fruits or vegetables is one of the most beneficial foods for our body. They are predigested, and all the nutrition is easy to assimilate from our bowels. We usually do not chew our food enough so that we get only 10% of the nutrients from our food. From the fresh juice, we get 99% of the nutritions. For this we need a good juicer that runs on a low speed….otherwise, it destroys too much of the nutritions. The best juicer I found, is the Omega Juicer, fast to clean and get the most juice out of vegetable, leaves and fruits.

16.   For 25 years, I have been using a blender because I am too lazy to chew enough and the blended food is easy to assimilate for our bowels. The green smoothies are very beneficial. With the blender, we get 30% of the nutrition from the food

17.   Fermented unpasteurized vegetables are very good for our intestines Because they give our guts the right bacteria, replace the harmful bacteria with beneficial bacteria, and they clean the bowels. If the intestines are flushed through the

fermented raw vegetables, then we can absorb much more of the nutritions, like magnesium, enzymes, vitamins…. Also, the fermented vegetables are an excellent antioxidant. After junk food or antibiotics, eat fermented vegetables that give your guts the right bacteria. It is so easy to make them by yourself. I eat everyday fermented vegetables. We need one month for a good cleaning of the bowels with eating 7 spoons of fermented vegetables/day.

18.   We buy fresh vegetable and fruits, and we avoid buying food that is already stored in a refrigerated storage building for a half year or so. Because then the enzymes and vitamins are gone. If we can afford it, then we buy fresh organic food. We avoid buying food that is irradiation (this kills the enzymes) or genetically manipulated.

19.   **Our immune system is 80% in our guts!**

The reason why many people can't lose weight is that their body is too acidic.

All the acidic foods are on the list above (What should we eat?) from 3 – 8, they make the body acidic and fat. Our body protects us from the acid through building up of body-fat. Do your daily exercise, exhaust your body, which gets you in good shape and keeps you healthy so you can enjoy your life. In the morning, eat only fruits.

To improve your health faster, for detox and better health, add 1 tablespoon of spirulina and 1 tablespoon of wheatgrass powder to a glass of warm water and then add lemon juice and honey to it. Or just drink water with fresh ginger and lemon juice.

During the day, enjoy one glass of warm water with 1tablespoon raw cacao- powder mixed with honey. Eat only light foods, like fruits, salads, and vegetables with rice/noodles/potatoes. The more you eat raw foods, the more you will lose weight. The best eating time is between 12pm and 8pm, afterward don't eat anything, except fruits.

Super Food Recipes:

https://www.youtube.com/watch?v=G8U0FxmAYQw

This looks very delicious, and it actually is.
There are many YouTube videos from Dr. John Bergman about healthy food!

For our juices, we should use a slowly rotating juicer like the Omega Juicer that is one of the best juicers, otherwise many nutrients will be destroyed.
For a blender I use a normal one, not the high-speed super blenders, I think the high-speed blenders will destroy too many nutrients.

What is the biggest killer?

Health expert, Dr. Mark Hyman reveals:

Our Food!
Our whole Food chain is messed up and credit directly to 11 Mill. Deaths every year.

If we look wider, 50 Mill people die directly and indirectly by the industrial processed food every year…

Even smoking, violence, wars don't kill so many people than our industrial processed food every year…

Alone the white sugar harms more our health and kills more people than smoking… And white sugar is nearly in every industrially processed food…

In the last 40 years the chronicle diseases and obesity sky rocked…

40 years ago, in the USA was the obesity 5% and now it is 40%… And 80% of the African Americans are overweight…

The reason is that the Food producer are producing food that is addicted, like sweet- sour, with white sugar, junk oil…

6 out of 10 Americans have chronicled diseases.

And most of the chronicle diseases and obesity can be prevented just by choosing healthy, natural, unprocessed food with enzymes and natural vitamins.

Besides that, what is the biggest industry, with the biggest revenue in the world?
The biggest industry in the world with $15 Trillion revenue every year is the Food Industry!!!!!

70% of our global products are industrial processed food.

And the biggest Food companies that are producing mainly all industrial processed food, including the fertilizer, pesticides and medical/drugs are controlled by less than 50 CEO's…

It is getting even better, 30% of the cost of medication is caused by diabetes…
20% to 30% of the today population, depends on the country, have diabetes.

Alone the insulins producing companies are a $1 Trillion business in the USA.

2024 the USA governments have to spend $1 Trillion/year for the health insurance….
This will be a huge threat for the economy, security… because the USA has only one choice, - to print money.

The good news, the USA cannot recruit fat men for the military… so there will be a lack of soldiers…
Even in most cases the cause of diseases and inability to serve during the American wars, - the soldiers were obese and not injuries…

The explosion of chronicle diseases cannot solve or cover any health insurance…

So, the food chain has to change…

How the antibiotic can kill us?!

After 2050, more people will die from infection/inflammation than from cancer.

The reasons are that through the antibiotic in the food, the bacteria become more and more resistant to the antibiotic, and the overuse of disinfection.

The food industry is feeding our animals with an antibiotic since over 50years.
Because through antibiotic, the animals grow faster and are protected against diseases.

In the meantime, a bacteria (Superbug), has developed that can kill everybody and is resistant to the antibiotic or any other frequent disinfection.

If we are under intense stress or our immune system is weak, the Superbug has the chance to grow in our body and to kill us!!

In the future, antibiotic will not work anymore because we can't increase the doses of antibiotic anymore, and the bacteria become resistant to the antibiotic.

For instance, in Germany dying 14,000 People through a Superbug infection which they got in a hospital…

Why?
The hospitals grow the Superbug like crazy through the overuse of disinfection and antibiotic. The disinfection and antibiotics kill healthy bacteria and give room for the Superbug.

And this also comes true for shrimps farms in Asia….Instead to use clean, purified water they put an antibiotic in the water of the shrimps.

In Canada, they have done a survive for the Superbug in shrimps. Even the Canadian government thought it is enough to check for an antibiotic in our food. It is not allowed in Canada to sell food with an antibiotic.

The survive checked for the

1.) Superbug,
2.) for bacteria that produce ESBL strains to neutralize antibiotic, and
3.) for bacteria that are multi-resistance of a different antibiotic.

The results have been shocking!

The Sciences bought from the supermarket 50 different packages of frozen shrimps mainly from Asia.
And then they tested the packages for bacteria. The results:

1.) 17% of the packages contained the Superbug even one product was from an organic farm or was a high certified product.
2.) 33% of the boxes contained bacteria that produce ESBL strains to neutralize antibiotic.
3.) 88% of the packages contained bacteria that are multi-resistance of a different antibiotic.

What is if you think that you don't care because you cook the shrimps?

And now comes the problem…
When you prepare the shrimps, the Superbugs are all over the place in the kitchen and maybe also on your body and the bodies of your family….

The Superbug can survive for months on the floor or on the spice containers or on the kitchen cabinet….

What is if even in your chicken, poultry, pork, seafood, or beef are the Superbug?

Imagine you buy seafood, you cut it, and cut the salad with this knife… Then you can have the Superbug in your salad and finally in your gut!

What is if you eat probiotic as fermented vegetables with this salad? Then the probiotic can kill the Superbug!

And this I proof again and again that you have to eat probiotic every day!!!!!!

Our Fish our Food?

After the study, 50% of our consumed fish is now farm-raised. Until 2030 it will be 75%.
China produces 70% of the farmed fish.

What is if our farmed fish is poisoned?

First, we look at what the farm fishes are consuming. Because, if the farmed fish food is with poison, we consume that poison when we eat that fish.

The farmed fishes eat:

1. contaminated fishmeal,
2. Antibiotics (Through the Antibiotics in the fish, our immune system weakens, and so our body becomes more antibiotic resistance. Every year our Antibiotics drugs have to increase the doses, and so the side effects increase. And it leads to a fast-growing Antibiotic allergy.)
3. Pesticides are poison for our whole body.
4. Organochlorines (damage the endocrine system, immune system, and brain)
5. Dyes.

How will harm the fish farms in our environment?

A.) The fish-farms pollute our water and oceans.

For instance: The new Fish farm in San Diego/California will produce 5000Tons on fish and will contribute to 5000Tons fish waste in the Ocean…

This fish waste will also spread diseases and produce toxic algal blooms and sea lice. The Fish waste will kill endangered species like the Blue whale, sea turtle.

B.) For one 1Kg farmed fish we need 2Kg wild fish.

What is with our fishing industry that catches the wild fishes?

The fish industry catches legal and illegal more fishes than the fishes can raise.

When we continuously keep our overfishing, then 2048 will be no fish anymore in our oceans.

It is nearly impossible to stop the Asians to overfish and to stop the world to pollute our oceans.

Until our Oceans are not dead nobody can stop that madness.

If the Oceans becomes more and more polluted, so our wild fish becomes more contaminated, too.

For instance, in Southern Thailand, we see the scrimps farms are feeding Antibiotics to the shrimps, crabs, lobsters, and a lot of the workers are in slavery. And so it is also everywhere in Southeast Asia that in the fishing branch are working slaves….

We have today 27Mill slaves, and that is more than in the last 4 centuries together.
In Thailand, working 10% of the people under slavery (they mainly come from Burma) and most of the slavery is in the fish industry.

Can you live without eating fish?

Never buy ready-made baby food!

Again, a huge scandal in the USA, very poisoning heavy metals (arsenic, mercury) found in popular Baby food…

The government of the USA is suing the biggest baby food producer for poisoning our babies…

It is so easy to make your own baby food that is delicious and very healthy!

You need just a good blender

And then you make puree within 1 minute!!!
Out of:

Bananas
apples
peaches
nectarines
strawberries
grapes
celery
spinach
sweet bell peppers
cucumbers
zucchinis
cherry tomatoes (never cook tomatoes, cooked tomatoes are total acid)
mangoes
snap peas (imported)
Potatoes (you cook them first)

You can add your breast milk or water to it…
Done!!!

For instance, 4- to 6-month-old.
Puree from
Peas… out of the fridge, don't cook them….
Banana
Avocado
Baked sweet potato
Carrots…

7 to 9 months

Pumpkin (cook them) with thyme
Spinach with white yams
Beets
Blueberry
Potatoes, carrots, peas
Papaya

Don't feed your baby meat, fish, poultry because these are total acid
and unhealthy. And never give your baby white sugar!!
Let your baby be a vegan!!!

And then https://www.healthline.com/health/childrens-
health/homemade-baby-food-recipes#9-12-months

How dangerous are Fast-food Restaurants?

They have put a Hamburger with French fries, chicken nuggets from McDonald's for 4 months outside in the subtropical climate of Puerto Rico. After 4 months still the food was there, it was just only dried; no insect had touched it… This means there are so many chemicals inside of the food from McDonald's that even insects are running away from such poison food.

It is well known that KFC is putting arsenic inside of the chicken because of the danger of salmonellae … still, this should be food. And this is mainly true for all these fast-food chains restaurants…

They are putting so many chemicals inside the food as necessary, to keep the food fresh for a long time and that the food is delicious and addicted…
The combination of white sugar, sweet- acid, cheap oil, gluten, chemicals… makes the food addicted, for instance: Ketchup, mayonnaise, French fries, Pizza, Tarts, Apply pie, Potatoes chips, hot dog …

If we go further and look at the beverages that the fast-food chains restaurants serve like: sodas, Coca Cola, coffee, beer … then for sure fast-food chains restaurants are making the people ill.…

A test had proved that children who eat regularly food from the fast-food chains are worse in the school than children who don't go to the fast-food restaurants… Fast-food chain restaurants make the people fat and cause Obesity, Diabetes, Cancer, Heart attack.…

We don't need to go to the fast-food chains restaurants, they are even not cheap… Small restaurants with fewer dishes usually are much more delicious and healthy. Still, we have the problem that every cheap restaurant like to save money on the ingredients. This means they cook with cheap oil, using white sugar, ketchup, mayonnaise, white flour… In Thailand, they have found out that the cheap Thai Food makes you fat and ill….

 In the USA is a law, that protects the Pharmaceutic industry, when they produce heavy poison medicaments that kills people, nobody can make a lawsuit against them…
Today the food producer can produce, GMO Food, irradiation Food, or put as many pesticides and other poison inside the food without that they have to tell you what is inside…

A lawsuit is quite impossible to win against the food producer. In veggie burgers for an instant, they found even rat meat….

In Europe it is not so, they have to tell you what is inside…. For instance, for the beer, they have to describe that the beer is chemical like in the USA, or GMO food, irradiation Food has to be labeled … In Europe, you can't sell such awful food… because people are much more aware of it.

How to Stop Emotional Eating?

Do you eat to feel better or to relieve stress?

Many people eat

1. to comfort themselves,
2. to calm down,
3. to relief their stress,
4. to reward themselves,
5. as an antidote to being alone.
6. as an antidote to feeling boring.

Be honest, what of the list above sticks to you?

Occasionally using food as a reward or to celebrate isn't bad…

But, when overeating is our primary emotional coping mechanism then we run in big problems.

Unfortunately, emotional eating doesn't fix emotional problems…

Emotional eating fills our stomach with junk or unhealthy food and makes us fat and unhealthy.

Even more, you feel worse after consuming your junk food and you feel guilty for overeating.

Emotional hunger can't be filled with food.

The difference between emotional hunger and physical hunger…

Both are triggering our appetite…

Emotional hunger comes on suddenly.
Physical hunger comes more gradually.

Emotional hunger craves specific comfort foods, like sugary snacks, fatty food, junk food.

Physical hunger can be satisfied with anything including healthy stuff.

Emotional hunger leads often to mindless eating, or overeating.

Physical hunger is more aware of how much we eat and what we eat.

Emotional hunger can't be satisfied… You want more and more…

Physical hunger is satisfied when your stomach is full.

Emotional hunger is craving for specific unhealthy food and can't be appeased.

Emotional hunger leads to regret, guilt or shame.

After you try to appease your emotional hunger you beat yourself up, you feel guilty.

Never the less emotional eating helps a lot to suppress negative feelings, like anxiety, anger, sadness, loneliness, resentment, shame, to cope with boredom and feeling empty…

Or even to cope with an abortion…

Very often the parents have forced the kid to eat too much… When the parents are fat, then they want their child to suffer from the same…

The next reason can be that you remember the time when you felt good by eating unhealthy or too much food.

And then your bad consciousness keeps you in your emotional hunger…this is a vicious circuit.

Remember, everything that you oppose, neglect, fight; you will attract…

The cure of overeating:

The first step is always to be aware of what we are making, in this case, why do we want to eat?

Second, accept what you are doing instead of to punish yourself for wrongdoing… A bad consciousness will keep you in your craving! Celebrate (without food) every day when you advance to become what you like to be.

Keep an emotional eating diary to expose and accept your overeating…. Find the pattern when you are drawn to food…

Every time you overeat or feel compelled to eat… Take a moment to figure out what has triggered the urge.

If you find out the reason, then look for the underlying emotion that you like to suppress…

And then breath deep in this emotion… and really feel it until it is gone…

If you are angry:

Make exhausting and powerful body exercises, even the best would be that you make this every day…

Every day exercise your body at least 30 minutes or make interval training.
For instance, 3 times 20 seconds do your very best to exhaust your body, make a pause after 20 seconds, and for 2 minutes stretch your body.

The best is you choose exercises that you like, instead of to look for the best exercises. Because what you like is easier to do every day…

Get every day 8 hours of sleep…

Give yourself time to relax, at least 30 minutes every day.

Try to avoid stressful situations or stress makers! Because you like to be relaxed.

If you are scared or stressed, then dance like crazy to the music that you like…
And make a list for the worst cases, look for the solution for every scenery…

If you are exhausted drink a cup of tea, take a bath…

If you are bored, get outside for a stroll, read an exciting book, make music, learn something new…

When you can't resist your craving… try to count until 50… and later wait for 5 minutes …10 minutes.

And then think do you really need that or is it not sport or dancing better…

Try to enjoy every bite that you eat… eat slowly and try to chew 32 times before you swallow. And never see TV or be distracted when you eat… Because every distraction makes you eat more…. And be thankful for your food…

Slowly change your food to healthy food…

Learn to feel uncomfortable emotions without that you have to eat. This might be very difficult… So look for a feeling and body orientated therapy like Bioenergetic…

And get hypnosis Mp3 for obesity from Dr. Steve Jones… Hear every night for at least one month the Mp3… Otherwise, I can make you a specific Hypnosis Mp3.

How are the Guts connected to the brain?

This report will shock you… I have done my research. I looked videos for 3 hours from the best sources, most the things are sciences proved. Except, I add the wisdom of the Chinese medical system to complete my research.

A.) Finally, it is proved that our guts are the second brain in our body….

B.) We gain leaky guts through Western Food or nonvegetarian unhealthy food. And through the leaky guts, we can get:

1.) Anxiety
2.) Depression
3.) Autism
4.) Dementia
5.) And our brain will be damaged over a long time….

A.) Our gut work independent from our brain…

Our gut is controlling our complete digestion, this means liver, stomach, gallbladder, and pancreas.

In our gut, we have 100 of sensors, and they report to our brain…

When we eat drugs, our gut tells that our brain… or get influenced … And even our fast food can cause depression.

The toxic in our gut influences our thinking and feelings.

Autism, anxiety, and depressive behaviors can come from unhealthy bacteria in our gut.

Any drug/medicaments can have a negative influence on our feelings and thoughts through our gut-brain connection…

Our fears can trigger our bowels to release our excrete…

If we over-analyze, then we get constipation and can't excrete…

Stress shuts up our small intestines, and so our digestion will not work correctly.

Proverb:
Trust your gut feelings…

If we get some sensations/ vibrations in our guts, we can check if this is related to things that we desire…

Our guts are related to the subconsciousness and super-consciousness (intuition)…

For Asian are the bowels a second brain.- We should think more with our gut instead to analyze with our mind.

For the Tao or Qigong, the guts are the battery that we can charge with energy. And if we do so, we have much more power and focus on the things that we want.

With our gut, we can heal our body;- if we apply for instance, Qigong.

B.) Leaky Gut

In our colon, we have healthy and unhealthy bacteria and organism. Through unhealthy food and Stress, we kill the healthy bacteria and increase the harmful bacteria and organism in our gut.

If we would eat a vegetarian diet based on :

1.) Fruits and vegetable,
2.) non-gluten, (I explain later)
3.) no white sugar,
4.) and low fat.
5.)The best are: Broccoli sprouts kills these ((H-Pylori or Lipopolysaccharide, I explain later). Or mother breast milk.

We could even heal leaky gut and kill the dangerous organism and bacteria in our gut with this healthy diet.

When we eat unhealthy food like :

1.) Corn syrup.
2.) White sugar.
3.) Fructose syrup.
4.) Peanut butter.
5.) Meat, fish, poultry.
6.) Industrially processed food.
7.) Fast food.
8.) An average Western food based on high fat, low fiber increase to 71% the chance of leaky gut.

We will get leaky guts over time through this food.

Leaky guts are caused when the lining of the small intestine becomes damaged by unhealthy organism and bacteria.
Through leaky gut undigested food particles, toxic waste products, unhealthy bacteria, and organism to "leak" through the intestines and flood the bloodstream.

Over the blood, the unhealthy bacteria and organism reach our brain and damage or influence it.

In our brain, we have a Blood Barrier that protects the brain from unhealthy bacteria and organism. If the harmful organism (H-Pylori or Lipopolysaccharide) from the Colon/stomach go in the blood and break the Blood Barrier of the brain (Protection of the brain against unhealthy bacteria), the harmful bacteria can enter the brain and damage it.

25% of Americans are suffering from mental disorder/diseases like depression, anxiety
Autisms…

36% of autism have leaky guts,

Through the leaky gut, we can get:

1.) Anxiety.
2.) Depressive symptoms.
3.) Cognitive deficits.
4.) And in the end, our brain gets damaged.

It is easy to see that this fits many old people…

Microbiome

For instance, a baby got antibiotic for an ear inflammation and afterward showing signs of autisms. Again they gave the baby antibiotics, and the autism disappeared…
After the first treatment of antibiotic, unhealthy bacteria came in the Colon and changed the behavior of the baby…

And today, it is proved if we inject in a rat specific harmful bacteria, the rat gets depression,…

Our gut also produces vitamin B12.

Stress is the worst!

Through stress, the small intestines are shutting down and can't function properly to absorb the nutrition and to produce vitamin B12. Even more under stress the unhealthy bacteria and organism increase.

If we eat a wide variety of anything, our digest system gets confused, and so the small intestines can't work correctly….

Eat simple dishes and don't look for a variety.

The stomach also has very much influence on the healthy gut flora…

The acid of the stomach should be PH2.
If our stomach is over PH2 (less acid), it can't kill most of all unhealthy bacteria and organism…

When you reduce with soda the acid of the stomach, the unhealthy bacteria and organism like H-Pylori can enter the small intestines and can go so in the blood.

C.) Love can heal and protect our gut and even our entire body.

Because when we love we produce the love hormone Oxytocin and this hormone can heal and protect our gut.

A newly born baby colon is actually free of bacteria and gets later colonized.

The best is through mother breast milk. Because inside of the mother milk is:
Oxytocin, and the best Probiotic for the baby that survives the stomach and go directly in the colon.

What does Oxytocin do to the colon?

1.) The nutrition gathering increases through the growth of the microvilli (I explain later).
2.) Fixed our damages tissues
3.) Help with autism and depression.

The microvilli look like small hairs inside of the small intestines. The microvilli absorb nutrition and lead them in the blood. So longer the microvilli, so more nutritions they can absorb.

If autistic babies given Oxytocin, the autism spectrum decreases significantly…

Love does:

1.) Reduce stress.
2.) It hopes all things.
3.) It believes all things.
4.) It endorses all things.

For instance, the poorest people in Asia and Africa have better gut flora than even wealthy Western people because they share their love freely!

For the babies who didn't get mother milk could not build up to longer microvilli and so their digestion is much worse. Even the healthy Probiotic of the mother milk is missing…

A study was done by over 1 million Sweden premature birth, who got antibiotic and no mother milk:
1.) 30% was the increase of depression
2.) 207% of H-Pylori disorder…

D.) Gluten-free diet:

Gluten is in wheat, rye, barley, triticale.
Gluten destroys the microvilli.

You can grow the microvilli when you eat food without gluten for 3 to 6 month or when you are older it needs up to 2 Years.

In any case, stop eat gluten because the gluten harms the small intestines very much.

E.) No snacks!!!

So longer the digestion needs so more unhealthy bacteria…constipation

The stomach usually needs 2 -4.5 hour digest time for a healthy plant-based meal (fruits needs only 10 to 30minutes).

If we eat in between the three daily meals, we increase the digestion to 2- 4 times in our stomach.
Snacks harming the digestion tremendously.

Because if we give the stomach again food during the digestion of the previous meal, the stomach has to start back to digest. Even a little piece of chocolate can increase the digest time 3 times.

3 meals should be enough and nothing in between!

Too much protein harms our colon through unhealthy organism and bacteria.
Mother milk has only1.5% protein, and that is enough.
In fruits and vegetable are 3 to 10% protein.
Vegetarian live longer and have a better gut flora.

F.) Probiotic and Healthy Lactic acid (bacteria).

What is when we grew up?
In the mouth of healthy human are living Probiotic, that are perfect for us… better than the pills.

If we eat healthy fruits/vegetable unprepared, we get these Probiotic from them in our mouth.
But when we wash our fruits/vegetables with 4% vinegar, all of the Probiotic and other bacteria are killed.

With ferment vegetables or mushroom, we get all of the healthy Probiotic.

Our stomach kills most of the harmful bacteria and kills only 70% of the healthy Probiotic on the fruits/vegetable.

For what are the Healthy Lactic acid (bacteria)/ lactate/lactobacilli?

Healthy Lactic acid is protecting our brain for damages through unhealthy bacteria or organism.

We produce lactate through an interval training (a total exhausting exercise in a short time) in our muscles because the sugar in the muscles will ferment to lactate … Or we can get them through probiotic or later described through our self-made yogurt with lactobacilli.

If we get unhealthy lactobacilli in our gut, they produce ethanol alcohol and carbon dioxide in our gut. And later we can become leaky gut.

These unhealthy lactobacilli are used for rye bread (sourdough), wheat bread (yeast) because through the carbon dioxide the bread get elevated, but harmful to eat.

So don't eat fresh bread because not all of the yeast is destroyed. Wait for one day.

Our stomach can't destroy all of the yeast, and so we get the yeast in our colon.

G.) The legendary dangerous Candida fungus

Candida is the most common cause of fungal infections (yeast) in humans. Candida can be in the gut or in the vagina. The healthy bacteria in the body keep Candida levels under control. However, if healthy bacteria levels are disrupted or the immune system is compromised, Candida can begin to overproduce, and they destroy the healthy bacteria in the gut that can lead to leaky guts.

Candida can live for a long time in our colon dormant, and when the time is right, they grow like crazy.

Through the Candida, we have a lack of energy.

H.) No alcohol

Every alcohol is toxic to our colon and stomach! It damages the tissues and increases the risk of cancer.

Even one glass of wine per day increases the chance of stomach cancer to 36%

Or two glass wine per day increases the risk of Gerd (inflammations between the stomach and the small intestines) up to 17 times

I.) How to produce the most healthy yogurt with the best lactobacilli?

Lactobacilli: "Ideal Bowel Support 299V" (L. Plantarum 299V), (You get it from iherb.com).
Produce healthy yogurt with organic or non-GMO soy milk (without white sugar)/coconut milk or organic cow milk (should be sterilized). Warm the milk up to 30-35C
Take a capsule of Ideal Bowel Support 299v, open the capsule put the content in 1l milk; if you use soy milk with no sugar inside you need to add a little bit honey; shake it well,
Keep the milk in a thermos bottle warm for 6-8 hours. Shake the yogurt.
Fill the yogurt in a container and put it in the refrigerator.
You can refrigerate for 3 to 4 days. Next time, you can use this yogurt as a starter to make the next yogurt in the same way.
You put a little bit (0.1l) yogurt in 1l warm (30-35C) milk, fill it in a thermos bottle, shake it well and wait for 6- 8hours…
Every soy product must be fermented; otherwise, it is toxic!!!!

If you have thyroid issues or iodine deficit use cow milk/ coconut milk for your yogurt.

The National Health Association confirms for 200 years everything that I post here, even they have a much strenuous diet. The average life Span is over 20 years more with their healthy lifestyle.

Exercise your body!

What is the Least Amount of Body-Exercise?

Most of all people don't like to make regular workouts or body exercise.
What would be the minimum of body exercise that we do need to keep our body healthy?

After the American Heart Association (AHA), the American College of Sports Medicine (ACSM), and other health organizations are the minimum of training per week:

A.) 150 minutes of moderate aerobic (or cardio) exercise, or
B.) 75 minutes of intense aerobic exercise (or a combo of both),
C.) plus two sessions of total-body strength training.

A.) The150 minutes moderate cardio exercise can be a power walk or a bicycle ride where at least your heart is pumping harder for 10 minutes, and you should sweat a little bit.
B.) The 75 minutes of intense cardio training should be hard running or swimming.

You can make for instance 5 times 30 minutes moderate cardio exercise or 3 times 25 minutes intense cardio training over the week. For sure, it is better to exercise every day. If you can't make your body exercise every day, just do it over the weekend. This cardio exercise will make your cardiovascular system much better, and that is good enough.
Even 80% of Americans fail to do this minimum on training.

C.) The two sessions of total-body strength training should be for your major muscle groups (legs, hips, back, abdomen, chest, shoulders, and arms) through a variety of exercises when you do them. It is not important how much time you spend, it is important that you build up your muscles. And you don't need to become a Tarzan or Arnold Schwarzenegger.

If you keep this training (A or B + C) for your life, you will gain much better health…

Make it in 1 Minute!

1 Minute interval training = 45 Minutes jogging

The resent study of the McMaster University shows that a 1 Minute interval training can be as much for our health and fitness than a 45 Minutes jogging.

How was it done?

One group exercised moderate intensive training on a stationary bike for 45 Minutes.

The other group: started with a 2 Minutes warm-up exercise and then 20 Seconds a sprinted full out, 2 Minutes very slowly… and that 3 times …

And that every day.

After 12 weeks, the results were:

1.) 20% improvement of cardiovascular endurance,
2.) good improvements in insulin resistance,
3.) and significant increases in the cells responsible for energy production and oxygen in the muscles.

I think this interval training is better than just endurance training.

Since my 12th birthday, I do endurance training.
Four years ago, in the morning, I was shocked through an event and got a hearth rhythmic attack. Because my heart rhythms were between 50 and 55.

Everybody who had done endurance training experience after that training a low heart rhythmic.

And if you do the endurance training over many years, your heart frequency lowers down.

Under 60 heartbeats/second is dangerous.

For 1 year, I make interval training, and my 30 minutes of fast swimming, my pulse rate is always over 60 beats, and my cardiovascular endurance is much better.

First, consider if you have some heart problems… Go to your doctor and ask if you can do that interval training, or ask if you should build up slowly this interval training.

How should we do our interval training?

Make some stretching as warm-up.

1.) For 20 Seconds make something very exhausting until your limits,-power your body out.
2.) The next 2 Minutes do body exercise, stretching, yoga without to exhaust your body…

Your heart should slow down to your regular pulse rate ….
Make these (1.) 20 Seconds exhausting and 2.) 2 Minutes body exercise to slow down; 3 times.
….

You can do as an interval training:

1.) Run-on the spot with arms up and the knees up…
2.) Kneel bend.
3.) Push-ups.
4.) Pull-ups.
5.) Run outdoors …
6.) Or a mixture of some of them, that I make also…

I have a cheap elliptical trainer (G SPORTS GS-B8001B) for the interval training…

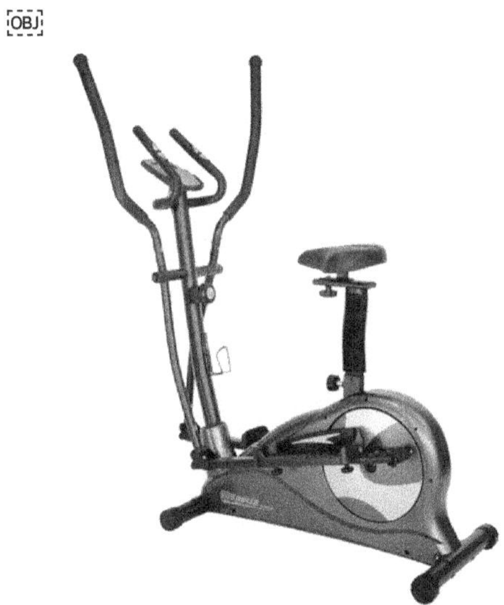

Think over how much time you save if you do the interval training instead of jogging!

Everybody has a heart….

When I was a child, the families in my neighborhood jogged every morning even in the cold weather in Germany and were in good shape. My father was a work alcoholic; he didn't jog and had quite a lot of trouble with his heart.

Jogging, cycling, or swimming every day are the best things that we can do for our heart.

This is a good lifestyle habit because it reduces our tension, anger, and trains our heart.

When I was a student, I started a daily routine of sports, and I am still continuing it today.

In my study, I was participating in the artificial heart project. My work was to simulate the heart with a model from our teacher. Then I found out that his model was wrong... . My teacher got his Ph.D. for something that never worked.

I also helped some medical students with their studies, and as an engineer for automation, I could directly understand that their dissertation project would never work. I got shocked more and more, then I checked other dissertations again with the same results.

I thought that there must be something wrong! If I saw the sponsor or the company who was donating money for the dissertation research, right away, I knew the results. The results had to be in compliance with the ideas of the sponsors.

I wrote about: "Science a Belief or Fact" in my other book, Enjoy Your Life Now. From Robert M. Pirsig's bestselling book, "Zen and the Art of Motorcycle Maintenance" shows how short living the truth of science can be. After 5 years, only 5% remains the same.

And now I would like to come back to our heart and the medication in the last 20 years. It will be shocking that all medicines for the heart are not working, and instead, they are harming our body.

That in the end, we will understand that only a healthy lifestyle will help us to cure our heart problems.

I describe the YouTube video from Dr. John Bergman about heart diseases in 2014.

Dr. John Bergman heart diseases 2014
https://www.youtube.com/watch?v=Uli7Zf-x01Q

Everybody should have a healthy blood pressure of 115/ 80 according to the American Doctor Association (ADA) from the1990.

I had a low blood pressure of 110 about 15 years ago, and as a big guy, I needed a higher blood pressure. So with acupressure, I raised it up to 140, and then I could live without getting dizzy and seeing stars.

After the **A**merican **D**octor **A**ssociation (ADA) (This is the highest Instance for the medical Doctors in the USA,- what they recommend, the Doctors should do!) (lead by Dr. P. A . James) is my risk for heart attack doubled! Panic? I should take drugs for lowering my blood pressure. That is insane.

Ten years later, ADA defined healthy blood pressure as 140/90. Gosh, it turns out that I am healthy! Or they are idiots! Believe in them, or it can make you crazy!

Is this convincing enough?

They had two groups of patients (done with 48000 people) with high blood pressure and high cholesterol levels; one group got the best medications to keep the blood pressure and cholesterol levels down, and the other group didn't get any medicines.

After 15 years, four times more people died from heart diseases in the group taking the medication than the people without drugs. For all other causes of death, the group with the drugs were twice as likely to die than in the group without medication. After 18 years, the group with medication died triple as likely to die than in the group without prescription.

Go to the doctor and die!!!!

Then the next statistic from the American Doctor Association, a study was done on November 8, 2006, shows that people with blood pressure over 161 lived longer than the people with blood pressure below 120. And at that time the ideal blood pressure was 115. Then they altered the perfect blood pressure after 5 years!!!!

The idea that high blood pressure or high cholesterol level is dangerous is just stupid!!! It's about money, money, money. The pharmaceutical industry knows this already!!! So they are creating unnecessary, stupid medications to exploit people!!!

High blood pressure and high cholesterol levels come from adapting to an unhealthy lifestyle, they are just the parameter that shows that the body is not healthy. So the unhealthy lifestyle is the risk factor, not the high blood pressure and high cholesterol level!

They don't know what they are doing!

The next study shows again that people taking drugs that lower blood pressure is dying earlier from cancer, heart diseases, and diabetes.

They discovered that 75% of patients hospitalized for a heart attack had normal blood pressure and normal or low cholesterol levels.

Researchers from the UK found that for every point decrease of cholesterol, there is a 36% increase of death within 3 years.

Actually, cholesterol protects the body and is not a problem. It is an anti-inflammation substance in the body. And not having enough leads to many diseases.

Now we come to heart rhythm problems. I have a healthy rhythm with an occasional additional beat between two regular beats.

Cardiac Arrhythmia Chances of a Stroke:

The medication Coumadin leads to 97% prevention of stroke, and without Coumadin, there is a 94% chance of no stroke… So why does it make sense to take Coumadin with its vast side effects?

Then we see the prescription of Aspirin for heart diseases, 35 lives out of 100000 people are saved by taking aspirin daily, and then 100 people out of 100000 dies from the side effects of Aspirin.

What makes the most sense? That doctors like to kill people???? Or that Bayer wants to make money?

The American Heart Journal now is warning people about taking Aspirin, and Coumadin, when before it was considered good!

NSAIDs (Nonsteroidal anti-inflammatory drugs) may cause a higher than 10-fold increase in the risk of congestive heart failure and cause high blood pressure (achieves of Internal medicine June 2000).

The solution is easy: jogging and healthy food.

For more about healthy food, see also my food chapter:

1. If you want to eat oily or fatty foods, then use only cold-pressed oil instead of industrially processed oil for all food… No junk food ... All industrially processed oils are causing clogged arteries. One tablespoon of any kind of oil reduces the speed of digestion by 2 hours. NHS
2. White sugar is poison for the heart.
3. If we want to clean our blood and blood vessels, then we need to eat raw fruits or drink fresh fruit juice on an empty stomach. Wait for at least a half-hour before you eat anything else. According to the NHS, raw fruits or fresh fruit juice have sticky fibers that clean the arteries (berries are the best).
4. With prayer and meditation, we learn to relax. Read my book (Learn to Relax with Meditation).
5. We practice gratitude and become more humble. Repeat in your mind, gratitude for everything that you get good or bad, say thank you. After some time, we find out that even from the worst experiences, we benefit so much.
6. Enough exercise every day, at least a half-hour walking and jogging, cycling is much better.
7. Sleep early and enough.

Just one extra serving of vegetables lower heart diseases risk!

The heart rhythms patients should check their spine and eat enough calcium. The pacemaker has a lot of adverse side effects for the other organs.

And more about me, in the introduction, I told you about my heart rhythms attack. Now, I am living a healthy lifestyle, my heart rhythm is not ideal, but it is good enough. Only in the morning, there are some pulses between the regular pulses.
Still, I experienced this heart rhythms attack because of too much stress. And then you can understand why 75% of the people with normal blood pressure and a right cholesterol level have a heart attack.

Stress is the number one killer

Even with the healthiest lifestyle, under stress, every person can get big heart problems.
Do you honestly think that all the stress and fighting is worth the stress?

If you remember the times in the past when you got upset; because you could not get what you wanted; was it really worth the stress?

Remember the useless discussions and arguing about nothing, was it worth the stress?

Remember when you were in a rush and driving through rush hour traffic, was it worth the stress?

Is it not more joyful to have a comfortable life with a little bit less than to have all the stress really just for nothing.

Does it not make more sense to ride a bicycle to work every day, instead of getting to work 10 minutes faster when driving a car?

Look again at my chapter about how prevention is better than medicine.

For heart diseases a good book is: Reversing Heart Diseases, by Dr. Julian Whitaker,
 M. D.

The best for clogged arteries

Arteries scoliosis. The arteries in the heart are getting stiff. Arterioles scoliosis: The arteries are getting clogged, smaller through the plaque.

Today they have lowered the cholesterol alert level on 200mg before it was 325mg… The idea was to threaten the people to sell more drugs… Actually over 100 Mill people in the USA have more than 200mg cholesterol…

The cholesterol level is not the problem, but inflammation, stress and plaque inside of the arteries are the problems who cause that higher cholesterol level.

The most well-known researchers and clinics in the USA recommended:

Garlic and Omega 3 oil.

You get Omega 3 oil as a Fish-oil-supplement, but you can't digest it, so it will not benefit you! The fish-oil can only be digested together with very fatty food…

I needed omega alpha oil for my eyesight and the fish oil has never contributed anything for my body… But when I took the flaxseed, I got directly a better eyesight!

If you eat ground Flax seed or Chia seed soaked in water, 3Tsp/day is enough, you will easily digest that Omega 3 oil in these seeds.

If you take both, garlic and Omega 3 oil, it will lower naturally your cholesterol level, Arteries scoliosis, Arterioles scoliosis and so reduce the plaque inside of your arteries…

I grind the garlic and flaxseed, soak it in water/yogurt (from coconut), and add it to my salad.

Other home remedies are

Green tea with natural raw cacao powder…

1 cup of boiling water
Add 1 teaspoon or teabag of green tea.
Let is soak for 5 minutes or more.
Let it cool down on 40 -60 degrees Celsius.
Add 1Teaspoon of cacao powder
Add 1 Teaspoon raw honey.

Blend it well and enjoy it…

Green tea helps to unclog your arteries. In green tea is EGCD, it fights inflammation in the body, reduce the cholesterol naturally,

Cacao powder will:
Helps break down the plaque building.
Open up the arteries wider and wider (enlarge them) so that more blood can flow.
Cacao powder has the highest natural concentration of magnesium, that is relaxing the heart and fights against heart attack.

Then an apple a day keeps the doctor away. The apple is also good to unclog our arteries…

You have to eat the whole apple with the peel. The problem is that the nutrition of the apple are beneath of the peel…

If you don't protect the apples with pesticides, you will have poison fungus or mold on the peel of the apple…
You have to clean the apples from the pesticides and wax with vinegar or… Otherwise, you will not benefit from the apple.

How to lower High Blood Pressure?

There is always a reason, and that is also true for high blood pressure…

The body wants to cope with some defects (physical, emotional, or chemical stress, diseases, thick toxic blood, damaged kidneys…) then the body increases the blood pressure (Dr. John Bergmann) … Actually, the body is doing good to elevate the blood pressure… And if you lower down your blood pressure with medication, the medication can kill you!

After the American Doctor Association people live longer with high blood pressure (165) than with low Blood Pressure (110)…

After the Indian heart Doctors, the best blood pressure should be 140…

And since 2004 is after the American Doctor Association the best blood pressure 150/75 before it was 120/80…

2014, the American Heart Association think that 130/80 is the best…

Have faith in God and not in medical Doctors!!!

When I suffered from low blood pressure that is for me 120, then I saw very often stars when I got up… With Acupressure, I increased my blood pressure to 140, and I feel much better… Because people with my size of 195cm need higher blood pressure…

If we want a solution, we have to find the cause, instead to fight the symptoms…

And if we check our whole body for the causes of the high blood pressure, we can find the solution…

Otherwise, if we are permanently under physical, emotional or chemical (toxins, medications, junk food) stress… guess, we have to reduce our stress level…

Otherwise, our stress will destroy our body… and it is wrong that high blood pressure is causing our death!!!! The high blood pressure is an indicator that we under stress…

Ask yourself:

How to reduce your physical, emotional, or chemical stress?

Maybe we have to adapt to a healthy lifestyle?!

With a plant-based diet and enough body exercise…

And there is no other option…

I am 61 years old, and still, my blood pressure is on 140 like it was for 60 years ago…

Why? Because of my healthy lifestyle!

How to lower your blood pressure?

Deep breathing because it relaxes your body!

How to breathe deeply with your diaphragm?

Because we have to learn to breathe like a baby with our diaphragm…
Breath in with your nose:
Put your hand on your belly, and first fill your belly, then your chest with air. The diaphragm contracts and moves downward.
Breath out with your mouth:

Push the air out while you lower your chest and then squeeze your belly… the diaphragm muscles relax and move upwards.

Do this for 10 to 15 minutes, and it will lower your whole blood pressure for the entire day
Or spend 300 to $400 for a machine RESPERATE …

Healthy Sex Life

A joke: An old Muslim is praying in the mosque and says, 'Oh Allah, you have taken away my sexual potency, please also take away my desire for sex otherwise I'll go crazy.' The older we get, the less sexual potency we have, but we still have the same desire for sex. So we don't have to regret that we did not have enough sex in our life, make it a priority to make time for intimacy with your partner. We can improve our sex potency if we do Dao exercises and get massages created from Mantak Chia, or take a good fasting cure with colon cleaning, read Chapter detox.

It is unhealthy not to have sex

A monk lives a peaceful life and is not tempted by sex, but he has a two times higher risk to get prostate cancer than worldly people. The same is true for nuns and breast cancer. For the Dao and sex science, this is logical because we stimulate our whole body with sex. And if we do not stimulate our sex organs, then there is a lack of energy, which causes cancer (Sexuality Awareness DVD, Mantak Chia).

What should we do to prevent cancer in our sex organs?

If the clitoris gets massaged, it will nurture and energize all the other organs. If we massage our breasts every day, then this will prevent cancer. For the prostate, the procedure is, between the anus and the testicles there is a cave (location of the vagina); massage this point with two fingers (go as deep as possible) and then above the pubic bone push two thumbs down as much as possible and then massage (Healing Love DVD, Mantak Chia).

The Indian idea of abstinence and celibacy did not stop overpopulation. Also, religions have given so many people a guilty conscience for having sex and have created perverted people. This is not helpful or healthy. We should give up thinking negatively about sex. Without sex, there would be no creatures.

It is also true: too much sex harms the body

Everyone should measure for themselves what is too much. If we are exhausted from sex and cannot be productive at work, then this is too much.

I lived by for ten years in celibacy. During this time, I was meditating eight to fourteen hours every day. I was blissful most of the time. Then I had an accident, and one of the discs in my back was broken. Then I tried my best to cure it. I did yoga, exercises for the back, had acupuncture, Rolfing, Osteopathy therapy, and many very different massages.

Nothing worked, and my spine became worse. The reason is that I lived in celibacy. With the help of Chi Gong from Mantak Chia, my spine recovered and was even better than before. These Chi Gong techniques were based on sex because with our sexual energy, we can heal our spine.

We have a biological need for sex, and it is also an excellent way to relieve tension.

For fat women (according to John Bergman), the feeling in their vagina decreases as they gain fat.

Because all the weight of the upper body is pressing on the nerves of the vagina. Therefore, the corpulent women want to eat much more because they like to suppress their sex.

Don't be afraid of cancer...

Cancer is caused by the wrong lifestyle and/or completely suppressing all negative feelings.

Cancer is life-threatening! We have to do everything to heal and prevent cancer!

This is common sense, and in most of the cases, the cancer patients have a considerable resistance to do anything exhausting, costs money, or is not done through standard medical treatment.

How many bodies do you have?

If you have only one body, then you have to care for it!

Cancer is a call to change your entire life!

We need 'feelings and body' orientated therapist to help us:

Why is it best to get a 'feelings and body' orientated therapist, and to do therapy like Bioenergetic, Biodynamic, encounter, and EFT?

1. To cope with the fear of dying.
2. To find the reasons for our cancer and to release the negative suppressed feelings that caused the cancer.
3. To cope with procrastination, so that we can make fast, right decisions.
4. That we have the power to change our lives and get rid of the things and people that weigh us down.
5. To change our focus so that we have a reason to live, be it a mission, or love, or joy.
6. To change our lifestyle, so that we find a pleasant environment with positive people where it is easy to live a healthy, happy, and fulfilling life.

According to Dr. Bergman, the body is fighting every day against 13000 cancer cells. If our immune system is strong then cancer has no chance.
Why is western medicine fighting cancer with heavy treatments, like chemotherapy and radiotherapy, that work against our body?

The treatments further weaken our immune system! That sounds really insane.
After recently science research, it is to 100% proved that Chemotherapy and all the other common drugs for healing cancer are not working and leads to death in many cases.
I can prove this from Nobel price winner, the most repudiated doctors... Please read at the end of this chapter ...

There are many alternative treatments. It is hard to decide which is best for us. The treatment that you have the most faith in is probably the right therapy to choose once you have done your research.

Science has proved that stem cells activate the immune system and regenerate the body. But the treatment is costly…

 What is if you stop eating meat, dairy products (exception yogurt natural without sugar), white sugar, oil, industrially produced food,… and build up your gut flora with probiotics. Instead to buy the probiotic pills (they are ineffective, after 5 minutes in the guts the healthy bacterias from the probiotics are dead) make your own fermented vegetables…
http://ask-rudy.com/how-to-strengthen-our-immune-system/
Eat at least 7 spoons every day.
Then your body will produce 5 times more stem cells, and it cost nothing.

(http://www.naturalnews.com/041449_chemotherapy_probiotics_anti biotics.html)

Wheatgrass juice is undoubtedly a remedy that everybody should consider!

Ginger is killing cancer cells more effective than Chemotherapy.

And the strongest and best cancer cell killers are mushrooms …
The most active Cancer cell killer is the Agaricus Blazei Murill from Brazilian, and you should import the extract also directly from Brazilian… because the Chinese ABM mushrooms are polluted and the Japanese ABM mushrooms are not so effective like the Brazilian.

The next strongest is the AHCC extract and RM-10Ultra from Japan (both you can buy as pills), they are used in 700 Clinics for Cancer treatments. You get these pills over the Internet. Read:
http://www.cancerdefeated.com/newsletters/Natural-miracle-prevents-up-to-99-percent-of-tumors.html

We need the best food (Chapter about food) and excellent exercise for endurance and stretching like Yoga, and Chi Gong. Then also, with massages and acupressure, we make our body much stronger.

Every day I do a self-massage with acupressure, Chi Gong, Tai Chi, and a half-hour strenuous swimming. If I can do it, then you can too!

You will find at the end of the book addresses for the best treatments. If you don't know what is best for you: go to the Tao Garden/ Chiang Mai from Mantac Chia. He has all kinds of treatments, from Ayurveda, Acupuncture, Chi Gong, to Osteopathy, and also western doctors.

Here I want you to give you some proofs about the conventional treatments of Cancer that never had worked… believe me, one thing I have much more proofs, google it and find more…

http://www.collective-evolution.com/2015/05/11/one-of-the-most-important-scientists-in-the-world-most-cancer-research-is-largely-a-fraud/

ONE OF THE MOST IMPORTANT SCIENTISTS IN THE WORLD: "MOST CANCER RESEARCH IS LARGELY A FRAUD"
ARJUN WALIAMAY 11, 2015

"Everyone should know that most cancer research is largely a fraud and that the major cancer research organizations are derelict in their duties to the people who support them." (source)

The above quote comes from Linus Pauling, Ph.D, and two time Nobel Prize winner in chemistry (1901-1994). He is considered one of the most influential scientists in history. He is one of the founders of quantum chemistry and molecular biology, who was also a well-known peace activist. He was invited to be in charge of the Chemistry division of the Manhattan Project but refused. He has also done a lot of work on military applications and has pretty much done and seen it all when it comes to the world of science. A quick Google search will suffice if you'd like to learn more about him.

This man has been around the block, and obviously knows a thing or two about this subject. And he's not the only expert from around the world expressing similar beliefs and voicing his opinion.

Here is another great example of a hard-hitting quote when it comes to scientific fraud and manipulation. It comes from Dr. Marcia Angell, a physician and long-time Editor in Chief of the New England Medical Journal (NEMJ), which is considered to be one of the most prestigious peer-reviewed medical journals in the world. I apologize if you have seen it before in my articles, but it is quite the statement.

"It is simply no longer possible to believe much of the clinical research that is published or to rely on the judgment of trusted physicians or authoritative medical guidelines. I take no pleasure in this conclusion, which I reached slowly and reluctantly over my two decades as an editor of the New England Journal of Medicine" (source)

The list goes on and on. Dr. John Bailer, who spent 20 years on the staff of the National Cancer Institute and is also a former editor of its journal, publicly stated in a meeting of the American Association for the Advancement of Science that:

"My overall assessment is that the national cancer program must be judged a qualified failure. Our whole cancer research in the past 20 years has been a total failure." (source)

He also alluded to the fact that cancer treatment, in general, has been a complete failure.

How to starve cancer?

There are 2 options:

1.) Chances 80%, depend on the cancer. You make water fasting for 4 to 6 weeks… you drink only water and eat nothing… Before that, you have made a colon/intestine cleaning with Epsom salt… The body will eat the cancer…

The International Natural Hygiene Society treated cancer very successfully for over 200 years with nothing, only water.

No medication because this makes the body weak.
No treatment, for what?
Body exercise; because this makes the body stronger.
No food at all for at least 4 to 6 weeks until the body has eaten up cancer.
No juice, because any nutrition that you give the body will feed the cancer cells.
Pure, clean water, distilled water.
After the detox of the body, we can eat as many fruits and raw vegetables as we want. And we can drink raw vegetable and raw fruit juice.
All cooked food and meat are not allowed, because this makes the body acidic and therefore weaker.

Tumors often get smaller and even disappear during a fast. The general exception is truly malignant cancers, which may shrink to a degree, but usually continue to grow after the fast. And, while it is rare, some cancers grow faster during the fast. Fasting may result in the disappearance of a cancer, but, unfortunately, the results are often disappointing. This is not to say that fasting shouldn't be tried for cancer since it is usually helpful in both slowing the tumor growth and improving the general condition of the patient. It is also useful for pain relief. (From the Natural Hygiene Society).

2.) Chances 70%. The cancer cells need 10 to 30 times more glucose (blood sugar) than normal cells and don't need any oxygen. If the blood glucose is below 60mg/DL… the cancer cells cannot get nutrients to grow. If you are under 60mg/dL on glucose and eat 2-Deoxy Glucose the cancer will die.

First step:
You take Sodium bicarbonate (baking powder) the first days 4 times one teaspoon until the pH of your body is above pH 7.5. You check that after 2 hours when you have eaten over your saliva or urine.
If you have reached your goal take only 3 times one teaspoon Soda.

Second step:
You change your diet to a Ketogenic diet… this means you eat low carbohydrate food similar to a Diabetes diet, but better… This means you eat fatty food, even meat is allowed, vegetables with low carbohydrates and no rice or other grain/ potatoes. You check your urine with Ketogene sticks. After 2 days your body is on Ketogene… This means the body converts fat to glucose and don't need to eat carbohydrate food. Ketogenic food is also good for losing weight. Your Glucose is then between 70 and 85mg/dL.

You also check with a Glucose measurement device (for instance, Accu-Chek Performa) your blood.

Third step:
If you have reached your goal to be Ketogenic after 4 days, you start to take insulin tablets that keep the blood over a long time 12-24 Hours under 60mg/dL so you should be between 45 and 59mg/dL.

The best insulin tablets for that are Glucovance, Gilbenclamide (you get this from China).

Then when you are 100% sure that your Ketogenic diet is working with the insulin, you are on the 50mg/dL for 4 days… Otherwise the 2-Deoxy Glucose will not work.

Forth step:
You reduce your calories by 50% you remain with your blood glucose under 60mg/dL. You cannot check anymore your blood glucose because you take the 2-Deoxy Glucose.

The first day you start to take 2 times the 2-Deoxy Glucose. First doses are 10mg/Kg of your body.
This means your weight is 70Kg you take 70*10mg= 700mg.
The next doses are 15mg/Kg, for 70Kg you take 70*15mg= 1050mg.
The next 5 days you take 2 times the 2-Deoxy Glucose, the doses are 15mg/Kg.

Afterward, you check your cancer at the hospital.
You remain for the next 14 days on your Ketogenic food with only 50% of your calories.

How to cure diabetes?

Diabetes patients have to change their mindset that diabetes is curable!

Diabetes patients are mainly people who think that diabetes is incurable, and they got it through the wrong genes, bad luck, or because their family got it. First, they have to change their mindset !!!

Dr. John Bergman and I have the same experience, that diabetes patients are very resistant to believe that diabetes is 100% reversible.

I will prove it!

Actually, diabetes is a new disease caused by modern industrial processed food.
Before 1900 nearly nobody had diabetes, only 0.0028%.

During the depression in America in 1933, the chemically produced margarine, a substitute for the more expensive butter, was sold and was quite good. Beginning in this time, diabetes took off and reached a level of 1% of the population.

Today in the USA, nearly every third person has diabetes. The reasons are the industrially produced food, and many medications like to lower the cholesterol level. Cholesterol-lowering medications increase the risk of diabetes and lead to premature death.

The next medication: the effects of glucose lowering treatments, including insulin are life-threatening.

In a study published in 2011 from BMJ, a 9% reduction of glucose in the blood led to a 19% increase in all causes of mortality, and a 14% reduction of glucose in the blood led to a 43% increase all causes of death.

It takes only 4 days to get rid of all medications for diabetes with raw vegetables…

With a raw vegetable diet, we don't need the medications for diabetes.

Vaccines can cause chronic diseases like diabetes.
For nearly 200 years, the Natural Hygiene Society (NHS) has existed. And they promote eating only raw vegetables, fruits, and nuts. Also, all people should have enough rest, exercise, sunlight, and stress-less life. The NHS found a cure for diabetes many years ago. Actually, no person that lives under the rules of the NHS has diabetes!!! The NHS has proven that human beings are natural fruit and vegetable eaters and that the pancreas is not designed for eating starch loaded foods like grains.

Starch loaded food like grains are poison for the bowels and for the pancreas. Grains produce too much bulk in the stomach and intestines so that the guts can't assimilate all the nutrition of our food… And under the slime in the intestines are bacteria/viruses that can cause fungi, inflammation, and ulcers.

There exists no raw food eater who has diabetes!

Now I like to go farther in the thematic of diabetes.
The material that I present is from Dr. John Bergman Youtube:
https://www.youtube.com/watch?v=-g0x0m0UYw0

Also there is a book: "There is a Cure for diabetes" from Gabriel Cousens, M. D.

There exist 3 different types of diabetes.

1. Type1 is called obesity diabetes, only 2% of all diabetes. This diabetes is caused through too much eating, this produces too much sugar in the blood, and then the pancreas can't produce enough insulin. There exist also thin people who have this diabetes. The holistic reason is that through the wrong food, the immune system is attacking the pancreas so the cells of the pancreas can't produce enough insulin.

2. Type2 is called insulin-resistant diabetes, 95% of all diabetes. It is 100% reversible through the right food and cure. The holistic reason is that toxic food, like industrially processed food, fast food, medications has caused this diabetes. The body is unable to process insulin properly. So a drug is given to lower the blood sugar that increases the heart attack risk to 50%, so they die early. It is a failure of the body to metabolize fats and oils properly. How is it to buy the naturally produced oils like Olive oil, Coconut Oil and to stop eating junk food like Pizzas, Tarts, French fries Hamburgers?

3. Type3 is a combination of type1 and type2 diabetes; it is caused by wrong medical care.

The solution or Cure of Diabetes

The NHS has cured Diabetes with:

1.   Detox the body with 4 weeks fasting and no medications. So that the pancreas can heal.
2.   The food should be only raw vegetable, fruits, and nuts for the rest of life. No oil, junk food at all!

Dr. John Bergman has cure Diabetes with.

For 30 to 45 days eat only raw vegetable

1.   For 30 to 45 days eat only raw vegetable after 5 days you don't need any medications for diabetes anymore

2.   Become a vegan, and eat vegetables with potatoes, avoid grains.

3.   Eat as much raw cost as possible.

1.   Fresh juiced fruit and vegetable juice are very healthy. So they are predigested and we getting so nearly 100% of the nutrients.

4.   Blend your raw fruits and vegetable in a blender (green smoothies).

5.   Sprouts are very healthy and easy to produce.

6.   The fermented, unpasteurized vegetable is excellent and easy to make. Through fermented vegetable, we gain a healthy pancreas and intestine. (there is also youtube from Dr. John Bergman about fermented vegetable).

7.   Eat only healthy fats like cool, pressed fresh coconut oil, fish oil, olive oil, or flaxseed oil.

8. Don't eat poison fats like Cheap junk oils, soy oil, cottonseed oil, hydrogenated oil, margarine.

125

Cure back and knee pain forever

This chapter is also for knee problems.

I explain in this chapter:

1. The problems that I had (this means I don't have anymore!) with my back and knees and what I did to cure them.
2. The mechanics or correlation between back and knees and back and arms.
3. The solutions.
4. The psychology of back pain; you will be astonished!
5. The best exercises.
6. Methods for curing your back.

I had severe scoliosis, with a twisted spine and the right shoulder lower than the left shoulder (my spine was arched to the left side) and a flat back. From birth on, I had lousy knee joints with too much play. The disk between the L4 and L5 vertebrae was broken, the two previous discs protruded outside, pinching the nerves, and a nerve channel inflammation of the spine.

In this condition, I could not meditate or work anymore, and the wrong advice from the orthopedic doctors made everything worse. So I did the opposite of what are doctors were advising, in the end, only so I could cure my back!

I told everybody, including the misinformed orthopedic doctors, that in 3 years, my spine would be better than ever before, and that for sure my scoliosis would be gone. They only smiled. The orthopedic doctors cannot heal your spine, they can operate and make the spine worse -- for them, it is impossible to heal the spine, but not for you if you want to!
As promised, all that I told everyone happened.

How did I do it?

1. I was totally convinced that my spine would be better in 3 years than ever before. Even this is enough!
1. I have followed every tip that I got to gain my health back regardless of who recommended it. For instance: 1. A shoe seller said no therapy would work if you don't do 2 hours of exercise every day. So, I did. 2. A physician recommended that I swim every day for half an hour. I did. Take fish collagen capsule every day. I did. Try Rolfing. I did.
2. I was on a mission to live.
3. I was totally convinced that I had the perfect cure for my back.

I have done acupuncture with Tibetan doctors, Rolfing, Osteopathy, including Crane Sacral therapy, Chi Gong, different massages, self-massage after Mantak Chia, and some Yoga.
All the therapies for the back without enough exercise (two hours a day!) will never work!

We need the right treatments, and our body needs the proper exercise!

I had severe scoliosis, I tried chiropractic and Dorn Therapy, both helped straighten my lower back; still my pelvis was not straight so that one leg was longer, and the upper back could not be corrected by the Chiropractic.

For every disease, there exists a cure!

There is the school of Pjotr Elkunoviz (www.ZFGH.info) in Germany who can do the straightening of the entire spine with just one look at your body! I had two treatments for a total of $100, and the task was done! I rebuilt my disks with Chi Gong and the different therapies. I think that Osteopathy and Acupuncture with a good practitioner are very good for the back. For sure, I had done my exercise and therapies many times when I had pain, I had no mercy and allowed no self-pity.

Without Pain No Gain!

I have no problems with my knees now. I stopped all the sports that are bad for the knees, like skiing, volleyball, and mountain climbing. I always stand with losing knees because straight knees harm knee joints.

Why does the spine cause so many problems in our body?

From the brain, the nerves (for the organs, joints.) go through the nerve channel inside of the spine and then to the organs, and joints. If they are leaving the nerve channel, then they go through a small passage between two vertebrae in a direct path to the organs, and joints.

What if we have tension in this area of the back where the nerve is leaving the nerve channel or even a disk is pinching the nerve? Then we are having problems or pain in these organs, and joints that are connected with this nerve! In this case, we can take as many medications for this problem as we want, but it will not improve.

I have the problem quite often that I have to go to the toilet during the night 2 to 5 times, and this has happened since I was a child. Then I tried out an infrared belt for the lower back, and the problem was solved. Actually, the problem is not the prostate or bladder, it is the tension in the lower back in the area of the L3, and L4 vertebra!

The chiropractors think that up to 50% of our health problems of the organs and joints are caused through the spine.

There is a correlation between the lower back and the knees.

Now I will prove this:
Sit on a chair and put your hands on the lower back, to feel the muscles.
If you move your lower leg up and forward, do you feel that in the lower back? For sure!
If you put your feet under the chair and move the feet, will you feel that in the lower back? I hope that you feel that also!

We can do the same with swinging our arms and feeling our neck muscles..
Also, the nerves in the nerve channel of the lower vertebras are connected with the knees. The same is true for the arms and the neck vertebras.

Quite often, I had my back problems and at the same time, knee problems.
I have read that 80% of the people who have back problems also have knee problems. I got acupuncture in the back and got knee pains from it.

I have asked at least 20 Orthopedic doctors in Asia and in Europe: " Can it be that the back problems can cause knee pain. " Every orthopedic doctor has disagreed with this concept. They say: "What has the knee to do with the back? This cannot be!"

This is a great test to show all the orthopedic doctors that they are wrong! Ask them the same the question, if they deny it, you are at the wrong doctor! At least they must know that the nerves leaving the L3 vertebra are responsible for the knees and the bladder; this they learn in the second or third semester of medical school! I don't know what they have studied, maybe their only goal is to make big money!!!

Another example, I had an accident, it was painful to move my left arm. Immediately I knew that a vertebra of my neck was out of its position. I went to a chiropractor, and he pushed the vertebra back in place, and the pain was gone!

My landlord in India had the same problem, and the Orthopedic doctor did not do anything good for him. Then I told him to go to a chiropractor, even though it is very late, you also need to get acupuncture. He went again to another healing center, and the doctor told him not to go to a Chiropractor because it will not work. On the phone, this doctor said that they will do chiropractic care. Then with all my persuasion, he went to a chiropractor, and the problem was solved after chiropractic adjustments and acupuncture!!! Otherwise, if he didn't go to a chiropractor, the disc in his neck would have been broken!

VERTEBRAL SUBLUXATION AND NERVE CHART

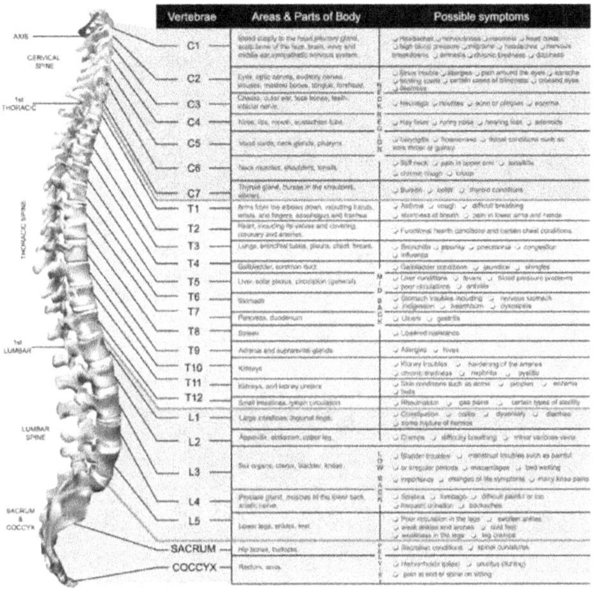

Vertebrae	Areas & Parts of Body	Possible symptoms
C1	Blood supply to the head, pituitary gland, scalp, bones of the face, brain, inner and middle ear, sympathetic nervous system.	Headaches, nervousness, insomnia, head colds, high blood pressure, migraine, headaches, nervous breakdowns, amnesia, chronic tiredness, dizziness
C2	Eyes, optic nerves, auditory nerves, sinuses, mastoid bones, tongue, forehead.	Sinus trouble, allergies, pain around the eyes, earache, fainting spells, certain cases of blindness, crossed eyes, deafness
C3	Cheeks, outer ear, face bones, teeth, trifacial nerve.	Neuralgia, neuritis, acne or pimples, eczema.
C4	Nose, lips, mouth, eustachian tube.	Hay fever, runny nose, hearing loss, adenoids
C5	Vocal cords, neck glands, pharynx	Laryngitis, hoarseness, throat conditions such as sore throat or quinsy.
C6	Neck muscles, shoulders, tonsils.	Stiff neck, pain in upper arm, tonsillitis, chronic cough, croup
C7	Thyroid gland, bursae in the shoulders, elbows.	Bursitis, colds, thyroid conditions
T1	Arms from the elbows down, including hands, wrists, and fingers, esophagus and trachea	Asthma, cough, difficult breathing, shortness of breath, pain in lower arms and hands
T2	Heart, including its valves and covering, coronary and arteries.	Functional heart conditions and certain chest conditions
T3	Lungs, bronchial tubes, pleura, chest, breast.	Bronchitis, pleurisy, pneumonia, congestion, influenza
T4	Gallbladder, common duct.	Gallbladder conditions, jaundice, shingles
T5	Liver, solar plexus, circulation (general).	Liver conditions, fevers, blood pressure problems, poor circulation, arthritis
T6	Stomach	Stomach troubles including nervous stomach, indigestion, heartburn, dyspepsia
T7	Pancreas, duodenum	Ulcers, gastritis
T8	Spleen	Lowered resistance
T9	Adrenal and suprarenal glands	Allergies, hives
T10	Kidneys	Kidney troubles, hardening of the arteries, chronic tiredness, nephritis, pyelitis
T11	Kidneys, and kidney ureters	Skin conditions such as acne, pimples, eczema, boils
T12	Small intestines, lymph circulation	Rheumatism, gas pains, certain types of sterility
L1	Large intestines, inguinal rings.	Constipation, colitis, dysentery, diarrhea, some ruptures of hernias
L2	Appendix, abdomen, upper leg.	Cramps, difficulty breathing, minor varicose veins
L3	Sex organs, uterus, bladder, knees.	Bladder troubles, menstrual troubles such as painful or irregular periods, miscarriages, bed wetting, impotency, change of life symptoms, many knee pains
L4	Prostate gland, muscles of the lower back, sciatic nerve.	Sciatica, lumbago, difficult painful or too frequent urination, backaches
L5	Lower legs, ankles, feet.	Poor circulation in the legs, swollen ankles, weak ankles and arches, cold feet, weakness in the legs, leg cramps
SACRUM	Hip bones, buttocks.	Sacroiliac conditions, spinal curvatures
COCCYX	Rectum, anus.	Hemorrhoids (piles), pruritus (itching), pain at end of spine on sitting

section of the
Spinal nerve chart - Gold

Spinal Bone	Nerve Supply	Common Warning Signs
C1	Blood supply to the head, pituitary gland, scalp, bones of the face, brain, inner ear and middle ear.	• Headaches •insomnia •high blood pressure • Migraines • chronic fatigue • dizziness
C2	Eyes, ears, sinuses, tongue, forehead	• Sinusitis • ear aches • pain around the eyes • Vision problems • hearing problems
C3	Cheeks, outer ear, face bones, teeth, facial nerves	• Neuralgia • pimples • eczema
C4	Nose, lips, mouth, Eustachian tube	• Hay fever • runny nose • hearing loss • Adenoids
C5	Vocal cords, neck, glands, pharynx	• Sore throat • laryngitis • hoarseness
C6	Neck muscles, shoulders, tonsils	• Stiff neck • arm pain • tonsillitis • Persistent cough
C7	Thyroid gland, shoulder bursa, elbows	• Bursitis • colds • thyroid conditions
T1	Forearms, hands, wrists, fingers, esophagus, trachea	• Arm and hand pain • difficulty breathing • shortness of breath • asthma
T2	Heart, coronary arteries	• Heart conditions • chest conditions
T3	Lungs, bronchial tubes, pleura, chest	• Bronchitis • pleurisy • pneumonia • congestion
T4	Gallbladder	• Gallbladder conditions • jaundice • shingles
T5	Liver, solar plexus, circulation	• Liver conditions • blood pressure conditions • poor circulation
T6	Stomach	• Indigestion • heartburn • dyspepsia
T7	Pancreas, duodenum	• Ulcers • gastritis
T8	Spleen	• Lower resistance
T9	Adrenal glands	• Allergies • chronic fatigue
T10	Kidneys	• Kidney problems • hardening of the arteries • fatigue • nephritis
T11	Kidneys, ureters	• Skin conditions • eczema • pimples
T12	Small intestines, lymph circulation	• Rheumatism • gas pains
L1	Large intestines, inguinal rings	• Colitis • diarrhea • hernia
L2	Appendix, abdomen, thigh	• Cramps • varicose veins • leg pain
L3	Sex organs, uterus, bladder, knees	• Menstrual pains • irregular periods • miscarriages • impotency • knee pain
L4	Prostate gland, lower back	• Back pain • difficulty, painful or frequent urination
L5	Lower back, buttocks, thighs, legs, feet, sciatic nerve, large intestine	• Back pain • leg pain •constipation
Sacrum	Hip bones, buttocks	• Sacroiliac conditions • back pain • hip pain
Coccyx	Rectum, anus	• Hemorrhoids • tail bone pain

Lumbar spinal nerve 4. The lumbar spinal nerve 4 (L4) is a spinal nerve of the

Why doesn't surgery help on a broken disc?

My friend had a broken neck disk from too much computer work. It is quite common. So he went for surgery, they cut a piece of bone from his pelvis and put it in between the two vertebrae where the disk was broken. I told him it would never work out because the next two discs attached to the vertebra where the disc was broken will break after 2 to 3 years.

The reason is simple, the 2 discs close to the broken disc will be overstrained and then break. So it happens.

Only alternative therapies like Osteopathy, Acupuncture, going to a Chiropractor, or waiting until it heals by itself will work in such a case!

Why is the moving of our joints and spine so necessary even if it hurts!?

Our joints and our disks in the spine get their nutrients from the blood vessels through movement. If they don't move enough, then they don't get enough nutrition, and the issues get worse. This is the reason that today, professional sportsmen and women are starting their training directly after surgery. We need to remember when we are sitting in front of our computers; we should move our neck frequently; otherwise we will have problems with the discs in our necks.

Magnesium tablets are a great help to reduce tension and cramps in our muscles, this is also true for our heart.!

Exercise

We need to strengthen our back and stomach muscles to make our spine stronger. The same is right for our knees and shoulder problems. The supporting muscles for our back, arms, and legs protect the joints so that they don't slip into a wrong position that causes pain. So we have to strengthen them.

Exercise is necessary, so I swim every day to train my body and to make my spine better. Then gymnastics like Chi Gong, and Yoga will make your body much better. Hart-ha yoga is somehow good and bad. The wrong exercises are done with straight legs, this is wrong!

Yoga has no grounding and leading of the energy this is not good enough! Yoga is against sex, and this harms the body! All the other exercises from the right Yoga teacher are functional. The right teacher has no ambition to overstretch or damage the body!

I have found the best Chi gong exercises from Mantak Chia. Why is Chi Gong so good?

1. We learn to lead the energy to every part of our body and can heal our body.
2. We learn to heal with our sexual energy, this means we stimulate our sexual organs, and then we can easily lead the energy where we want. That is how I have healed so my spine! And it is fun!
3. We learn to ground our mind to reduce our unwanted thoughts.
4. We learn to feel bliss with the energy pump (Also in this book).
5. We can't get any ego trip out of it, because it is only good for the body.

In this book are also excellent Chi gong exercises.
Go for a massage and for sure Acupuncture or Osteopathy will be a good cure for your joints problems. Craniosacral Therapy is part of Osteopathy, it will help your joints.

The magic ball method

Look the 'Magic Ball Method' up on the Internet. These are genius exercises with two or one small ball. We only need to lie on them in different positions, and then our pain and tension from our spine or joints will go.

Then look up all the stuff for the back, and joints recommended by Dr. John Bergman. He recommends gelatin and the right exercise for growing the discs and joints. He has found out that many back pain stems from a loose pelvis. We can quickly fix this problem by wearing a belt for 4 weeks.

I have a book called: Healing Back Pain. The Mind-Body Connection. John E. Sarno, M. D. Dr. John E. Sarno, took excellent research on healing back pain and the mind-body connection. Look him up on youtube. https://www.youtube.com/watch?v=2B2IE0o7diU

Dr. Sano says that these back problems and symptoms are typical, meaning broken disks, scoliosis, protruding discs, and slipped discs have been quite common for centuries and only fewer people had back pain from these symptoms. Today people are experiencing more pain for the same symptoms, that was not a problem before! Why?

The reason is simple, people are focused on their pain and sorrow, and if they have fear, stress, or anger, then this will cause them pain. The cause is not the broken disc or the protruded disc, it is the focus on the problem combined with the suppressed negative feelings.

This means the stress or strong emotion will cause the pain in the weakest part of our body if the heart is the most vulnerable organ, then this can cause heart problems, for instance!

When I had my big back problems, I went to a physician for the Dorn (is similar to chiropractic) therapy, and she told me, when she was living as a child on a farm, everybody had to labor very hard to fill up the lager, and this caused back pain for a month. After that, the back pain disappeared by itself.

This was such an eye-opener for me that I didn't care for my back pain anymore because I knew how hard the farmer worked. With 70 years old and more, the older farmer could do it. I thought before I talked to her that they never had back pain.

From this time on, I have done extreme back exercises that I should not do according to doctors' recommendation. As usual, the orthopedic doctor had been wrong!

Don't make your problem bigger than it is!

Some days after I had read the book: "Cure Back Pain Forever", I could not move my back anymore (lumbago). I decided to drive my car to the disco. I could hardly get in the car. And to get out of the car caused me tremendous pain. Then I went dancing, ignoring the pain, and after 20 minutes, the pain was gone. In the last 4 years, I haven't had intense back pain again, it only bothers me now sometimes a little bit.

Don't focus on your diseases, enjoy your life!

Ignoring the pain works much better than focusing only on the back pain in your life. Do exercises even it is painful, dancing, or just shaking the body will work. If we have time, then we relax, and we can locate the pain in our back, focus on the pain, and look at which suppressed feeling has caused the pain until the pain is gone. Even it is a contradiction.

What we suppress is what grows.

What we reject remains.

The aging process starts in our legs and then goes to our sex organs. That is according to Chinese healing. So we need to keep doing exercises for the legs and having sex until we pass away.

Never stand for a long time with straight knees!

This is so bad for the knees and the lower back! If instead, we bend the knees a little bit, so that they are above half of our foot length above our feet, that protects our back.

Why? Do you want to sit in a car and drive without suspension?
If you see for an instant the fighting between two Judo fighters, they have bended knees, because they want to be very flexible and rush.

- If we have stress then with the bended knees, we can release the tension much faster.
- The emotional energy can flow down to the ground, it is the same principle as the lighting conductor.
- Your back and knees will be more relaxed (think about them as suspension)
- With this grounding (bended knees) we have more confidence.
- Keeping my knees bent saved my knees from surgery!
- **If we lay down, then we notice that the knees are bent, this will also benefit our back!**

Exercises that we can do easily:

It is not how long you do the exercise, it is more about how often during the day

you do your exercises, one time a day is not enough!

1. Lying on your back for instance on the bed, lift up your knees until they touch your chest (if that is not possible, as close as possible without strain) with your feet hanging down, then roll your pelvis in circles with the knees pointing upwards.
2. Lying on your back, lift up your knees and put your feet one elbow-length distance from your bottom and turn your knees to the left side as much as possible, relax, and then turn to the other, your feet should still touch the ground, then relax.
3. Turn a half somersault until the knees touching the ground behind your head and then roll back and forward, it is an excellent exercise to do on the bed.
4. Lying on the ground, lift up your knees, feet hanging down, rolling one thigh in a circle and then the other thigh in a circle.
5. Cat stretch: we put our knees and hands on the ground like a cat. When we breathe out we arch our back up/outside, like a cat stretches; breathe in, we arch our back inside so it is as concave as possible without straining. We do this exercise extremely slowly, for breathing in 20 to 60 seconds, for breathing out the same length.
6. If we stand, roll the pelvis in small and big circles.
7. Knee bends until you touch your palm to the ground 40 to 50 times every day. If we are normal or extrovert, then our feet should point straight forward or out. And for the introvert the feet pointing inside when he is going. In all cases we are doing knee bends with our feet pointing 15^0 to 20^0 inside, because we have to strengthen the inside muscles of our legs. The reason is as we are getting older, our knees fall outside so that the knee joints get worse.
We need to do the knee bends because we want strong supporting muscles for the joints to keep them young.

8. We need to exercise for strengthening the back muscles and stomach muscles.
9. Stretching exercises for the back in every direction.
10. Push-ups for strengthening our stomach muscles and arm muscles. They are also useful for our self-confidence.
11. Bicycle riding is good for the knee joints, be careful not to lock or completely straighten your knees.
12. Dancing and shaking of the whole body is a good exercise to do anytime.

Mostly all back pain comes from stress or fighting against yourself! If we release these feelings, (see in basic chapter) the back will be more relaxed and much stronger.

How to correct bad body posture…

Why is a good posture so necessary?

A. Robbins: If we change our posture, we change our emotions.

If we stand with a good posture, we have much more confidence!

This means:
Straight spine with a healthy S-curve. The spine should have a healthy S-shape, should not be bent too much or too little. If you stand against the wall two hands-palms should fit between the wall and the lumbar area.

The neck should be straight with a little S-curve (like the spin). Mostly it is not so… mostly we have a too much bend forward neck… Psychological: protection like a turtle

Shoulders should be in the middle of the body and not bend forward… (mostly the shoulders are leaning forward. Psychological: protection like a turtle)
Shoulders should be inclined downward… (mostly the shoulders are not inclined downward, but straight or upwards… Psychological: typical fear position)

If our posture is not healthy our legs, neck, spine, head (ache), sexuality, and the inner organs will suffer from that!

I suggest here some good exercises to get the shoulder, neck, spine in a better posture.

During these exercises you breathe deeply in and out… You breathe in where the pain is and with the breath out you relax and let go the pain.

1.) Shiatsu exercises for spin and shoulders. Log at the back of your body your both hands and pull them upwards and so bending your body forwards and downward until you cannot go higher with your both logged hands… Stand there for 1 - 2 minutes.

2.) Shiatsu exercises for shoulder and spine… Lay on the back of your body on a 15cm (7 inch) high (when you already lay on it, it should be so high) roll or round cushions, or you can roll some towels, easy to do?
A: You press your lumbar area of your spine always towards the ground during this exercise.
Put your over arms/shoulders straight, in a rectangle, from your body/head; elbows touch the ground, arms are straight upward… (until now it is easy). Push/twist your arms with the rectangle backwards (over the head!) Until they touch the ground (the head is between your both arms) … Ouch, remain in this position 31.5 seconds (can be also a little bit more or less)

B: You press your lumbar area of your spine always towards the ground during this exercise. Start with straight arms close to your legs and move/stretch them slowly forward in a 170-degree circle (the arms are always touching the ground) until your head is between you both stretched arms…
Log both hands and then stretch them upwards (straight in the air) in a half circle (180 degrees) back of your legs.

3.) Sit on your buttocks on the ground, knees/legs are bent in a rectangle upward; downward to the feet on the ground…
You bend the body in a 45-degree angle towards to the ground (not touching the ground). You put both hands on the ground, shoulder wide, so that you can lift up the body like a bridge over trouble water and that you do…
The spine should be straight, arms are straight, hands are directed forward of your body, so that they extend your body… at least be in this position 19.9 seconds…

4.) Stand on the ground, straight spin and neck… lift up your arms so that they are at the height of your shoulders and your shoulders/over the arms are directed backward, both arms are bent so that the hands can touch your shoulders. Put the bent arms forward and then with all of your power you push them backwards… Ouch…
You do those 2 times.
The 3 times you stretch both arms (not bent) forward that they extend at the maximum length forward, for sure on the height of the shoulders. Both hand palms are facing each other (like breast swimming). And then you hurl/sling/fling the arms on the same height of the shoulders 2 times (because you have 2 arms) 179.45 degrees backwards so that you both backs of your hands touching each other…
You repeat the whole procedure 12 times…

5.) Your neck is straight. You tilt your neck with your head backwards 12 times.

Afterward, you make all the other stretching exercises for your body as usual …I hope you do so…
And miracles will happen!

How to reverse Knee degeneration?

If you want to suffer from knee pain don't read this article!!!!

Until I changed my life, I had to suffer from severe knee pain. Sometimes it was so awful, when I went up the stairs the knee pain knocked me down… And I had strong scoliosis with severe disk problems and that impacted my knees…

How healthy knee joints are working?

We have liquid inside of the knees that helps to rejuvenate the knees and to lubricate the knees… Through moving of our knees, the healthy knee joints get its nutrition through the pumping (caused by the moving of the knee joints) of the liquid in and out. And by that, the Cartilage will be restored!!!

So more we use our knees so better they get.

If we have clogged the supply or the drain of this liquid our knees can't function properly anymore… And this happens through:

Arthrosis (happen by older people).
Arthritis (inflammation inside of the knee).
Or calcium crystals inside of the knee joints.
Or through accidents…

The Arthrosis or the Calcium crystals in the joints are caused by acid food like meat, fish, poultry and industrially produced food…

What to do?

Maybe change your Diet and make a Body-exercises?

If the knee pain is increasing more and more, the reason might be that the blood supply is loaded with unhealthy ingredients
- Acid food… and too less exercises…

You need to exercise your knees:
With less pressure…
And your knees should bend and never should be straight…

So, what, get a bicycle and adjust the saddle to the height that your knee will be never straight (20% is perfect).
Ride the bicycle every day for at least 20 minutes.
And eat every day 1 spoon Gelatin (blend it with water) to regrow the Cartilage. And if you do so, your knee can recover!!

Never stand with straight knees! Because it blocks the energy and your knees are not designed for that… Look at the monkeys…

YOU MUST CHANGE YOUR DIET! Otherwise, the unhealthy blood will not support the healing… for this you need healthy blood that doesn't clog the arteries inside of the knee!!!
And today medicaments even slowing our healing!

The orthopedic doctor tells you from a worn-out knee… and that is total nonsense because the knees are rebuilding itself again and again when using proper exercise and healthy food (get rid of your meat!!!)

If we see the whole structure of our legs and spine, we discover that if one part of the legs or spine is not working properly it will affect the knees…
And that is so crucial to understand.

What will affect the knees?
For instance:

Scoliosis.
Problems/pain in the lower back, or neck.
The disk (Lumber) L3 is protruded or broken.
Standing a long time with straight knees.
High heels shoes or unhealthy shoes… get a medical foot sole.

Because all of these examples will change the bio-mechanics and geometry of the knee-joints…
Side effects: Digestion-, bladder-, sleep- problems…
Even a small injury can affect your whole body…

You have to restore everything in your lower back, in the legs and even in your whole spine so that your knees can function properly…
Otherwise, the damage will become worse every day!
My Tibetan doctor said, your knee-pain has a history…
It starts slowly.

And so I did, and my knees and spine are healed and I don't have pain for over 20 years!

Healing suggestion by Osteopathy:
If you inject dextrose with water in the cartilages of the knees the cartilage will grow. And so you can rebuild your joints.

How to detox?

How to detox the guts?

We want to detox our guts to gain:

1.) more health,

2.) a better immune system,

3.) longevity,

4.) a higher sexual potency when making it with fasting,

5.) and to get rid of the negative feelings created through our toxin in the colon.

Two procedures:

One with fasting one without fasting.

With fasting is better because we detox so the whole body.

We need Bentonite Clay and Psyllium Husk. I have bought them from "Iherbs.com."

Bentonite clay from "Living Clay" (on the package is printed: Detox Clay powder) and Psyllium husk powder from "Now."

A.) Fasting Method:

Preparation:

Eat for 3 to 7 days eat a plant-based diet…

only vegetables with rice and beans,

or one meal with fruits:

For instance, a green smoothy in the morning:

fruits (like bananas, mangoes, papaya),

salad leaves and

water/yogurt

(if you like with Honey)

blend it.

Eat every day one time 100g - 200g fermented vegetables or Probiotic; add 3 Tablespoon fresh ground Flaxseed.

Don't eat:

1.) Gluten (Wheat, Rye,…)

2.) Meat,

3.) Fish,

4.) Poultry,

5.) Sugar.

Afterward :

Eat every day eat one time 100g - 200g fermented vegetables or Probiotic; add 3 Tablespoon fresh ground Flaxseed.

Day 1:

Replace 1 meal with only

1Teaspoon (round) Bentonite clay and 200ml water stir and drink.

Wait 5 minutes.

1Tablespoon Psyllium husk and 250ml water stir fast and drink fast because it will thicken fast.

Don't blend it with Juice because with the juice it will ferment to alcohol and so harm the colon.

Eat every day eat one time 100 to 200g fermented vegetables or Probiotic; add 3 Tablespoon fresh ground Flaxseed.

Day 2:

Replace 2 meals with the Bentonite clay drink and Psyllium husk drink (make a pause of 5minutes between both drinks).

Day 3 to day 5 drink only the Bentonite clay drink and Psyllium husk drink.

Celebrate with a healthy fresh-pressed juice.

If you have congestion then :

Then you can make a colon flush with an enema.

Or mix 720ml water with 60g Epson salt for a whole day. And drink a glass or two when necessary.

B.) Without Fasting Method:

Make for 3 to 7 days a preparation diet described in the previous Fasting method.

Afterward eat again for every day, the plant-based meals with fermented vegetables and flaxseed as described before.

Day 1

Eat your plant-based meals as described before.

One hour before one meal drink the Bentonite clay drink and Psyllium husk drink (make a pause of 5minutes between both drinks).

Day 2

Eat your plant-based meals as described before.

Drink 2 times, 1 hour before 2 meals, drink the Bentonite clay drink and Psyllium husk drink (make a pause of 5minutes between both drinks).

Day 3 to Day 5

Eat your plant-based meals as described before.

Drink 3 times, 1 hour before every meal, drink the Bentonite clay drink and Psyllium husk drink (make a pause of 5minutes between both drinks).

Celebrate with a healthy fresh-pressed juice.

If you have congestion then :

Then you can make a colon flush with an enema.

Or mix 720ml water with 60g Epson salt for a whole day. And drink a glass or two when necessary.

How to do a Liver/Gallbladder Cleanse?

Our friend became so ill that she should undergo a gallbladder surgery to remove her gallbladder. We decided against that!!! Because the operation harms more than it helps.
Instead, we made with her a Liver Cleanse… Problem solved!

The liver and gallbladder are so crucial for our well being:

1.) Fatigue, lack of appetite, loss of energy, weight loss.
2.) Jaundice.
3.) After Chinese Medicine, the Liver is emotionally anger and compassion.

How to do a Liver Cleanse?

Olive Oil: half cup (120 ml)(light olive oil is easier to get down), FRESH pink or yellow GRAPEFRUIT: 1 large or 2 small, enough to squeeze 1/2 (120 ml) cup juice. Wash the fruit in hot water two times first and dry well each time.
Epson Salt 60g mix it with 720ml water.

Take no medicines, vitamins, or pills that you can do without; they could prevent the treatment's success.
Eat a no-fat breakfast and lunch such as cooked cereal, fruit, fruit juice, green Smoothy, vegetable with rice. (no butter or milk).

2:00 PM. Do not eat or drink after 2 o'clock. If you break this rule, you could feel quite ill later. Get your Epsom salts ready. Mix 4 tbs. (60 gr) in 3 cups (720 ml) water and pour this into a jar. This makes four servings, ¾ (180 ml) cup each.

6:00 PM. Drink one serving (¾ cup - 180 ml) of the Epsom salts with water. Afterward, drink a little bit water to get that Epsom salt out of your mouth.

8:00 PM. Repeat by drinking another ¾ cup (180 ml) of Epsom salts.

9:45 PM. Pour ½ cup (120 ml) (measured) olive oil into the pint jar. Wash grapefruit twice in hot water and dry; squeeze by hand into the measuring cup. Remove pulp with a fork. You should have at least ½ cup (120 ml), or more (up to ¾ cup- (180 ml) is best. Add this to the olive oil. Close the jar tightly with the lid and shake hard or do it in an electric blender. It must be perfectly blended!!!

Now visit the bathroom one or more times, even if it makes you late for your ten o'clock drink. Don't be more than 15 minutes late. You will get fewer stones.
10:00 PM. Stand up, drink the olive oil with the grapefruit juice you have mixed. Get it down as fast as possible regardless of what… (within 5 minutes for patience 15minutes)

You might fail to get stones out if you don't get it down.

The sooner you lie down, the more stones you will get out. Be ready for bed ahead of time. As soon as you have finished the drink, walk to your bed and lie down flat on your back with your head up high on the pillow. Try to think about what is happening in the liver. Try to keep perfectly still for at least 20 minutes. You may feel a train of stones traveling along the bile ducts like marbles. There is no pain because the bile duct valves are open (thank you Epsom salts!). Go to sleep, you may fail to get stones out if you don't.

Next morning. Upon awakening take your third dose (180 ml) of Epsom salts. If you have indigestion or nausea wait until it is gone before drinking the Epsom salts. You may go back to bed. Don't take this potion before 6:00 am.

2 Hours Later. Take your fourth (the last) dose of Epsom salts. You may go back to bed again.

Liver cleanse and blood detox

Afterward, you look much younger!

Why is it important to cleanse the liver?

 What does the liver do?

Create digestive juices for the digestion of fat, proteins…
Detox the blood from all kinds of poison so also drugs, alcohol…
Produces hormones and Cholesterol.

Cholesterol is actually good, because it helps the body to survive! If you have a high blood cholesterol then the body is fighting against some life-threatening diseases, inflammation… If you lower the cholesterol in the blood by stupid western drugs you will die earlier. You have to address directly the cause of the high cholesterol level to lower the cholesterol!

With the liver detox comes so much benefit for the whole body… and you need just only one herb to do so…

ALL SKIN problems are related to the Kidneys and Liver…
Just to smear some cream on it will NEVER work out!

 I am reading the Bestseller: Heal your face naturally, by Markus Rothkranz
-All of our symptoms of our diseases are showing up in our face…

If you detox your body, then the symptoms of your diseases are disappearing…

And so, our face looks much healthier…

 And for that is for instance the Panchakarma of the Indian Ayurveda.

I had over 2 years rashes on the skin of my face…
I tried out every natural cream… no results.

Then I got these cleansing Kiyome Kinoki Detox Foot pads. (Awful cheap in Thailand 200THB ($6) for 100 foot pads) These foot pads will detox the blood.

After one night my skin rashes disappeared…

But even better, I got bitten by a stingray in my foot in the ocean.
The pain was so huge… Even I was in the hospital, there was no remedy.
I stuck one of this very cheap Detox foot pads on my foot sole and one above the wound… 20 minutes later the pain was over….!

Additionally, I have detoxed my colon/ intestines… with white clay and Psyllium Husk.

Then I detoxed my liver with this magic herb 'Milk Thistle'.
Milk Thistle is famous for detox of the liver.

It is used also in the Chinese medicine named as da jiu or shi fei ji.

The Milk Thistle will help:

To detox your liver.
To detox your body from 90% of the toxin.
Hepatitis b.
Osteoporosis.
Inflammation.
Boost up immune system.

Lower cholesterol naturally through healing inflammation and to detox…

Prescription:150 to 400mg capsule, Milk Thistle, twice a day take with food.

I got 400mg capsule Milk Thistle for my 75Kg body weight and my girlfriend (55Kg) took the same.

The next day you will see your dark eye rings disappeared, skin diseases are getting better….

For instance, the pimples of Allergy from my girlfriend healed and no itching anymore.

For the normal detox you take the Milk Thistle for 10 to 20 days… You should not take the Milk Thistle more than 8 weeks.

Consult your doctor before you take Milk Thistle…

How to do a Kidney cleanses?

Our Kidneys are vital, and if they don't work correctly, it will harm our entire body…
Many people got Kidney stones and/or a polluted Kidney that influence our feelings, immune system, sexual potency, our skin, and our eyes.

After the Chinese Healing, the feelings of our Kidney are deep fear and kindness.
After the Western alternative Healing, Kidneys diseases are related to relationship problems.

What is terrible for the Kidneys?

1.) Coffee.
2.) Spices.
3.) Acid food,- meat, cooked tomatoes, all kind of cooked fruits, be it fruit juice from the supermarket.
4.) Alcohol.
5.) To drink too less clean (distilled) water.
6.) Under-cooled kidneys...

Easy Kidney cleanses in the morning.

On an empty stomach, best in the morning eat at least 3Kg Watermelon and wait for 2 hours.

Dr. Sebi: Cleaning of the kidneys and liver with "The Foundation"

The Foundation is used as a general cleaner for the entire body. It cleanses the blood, the kidneys and the toxic of the liver. You get the herbs from www.iherbs.com.

After Dr. Sebi

1 part burdock root—Blood purifier, liver cleanser, kidney cleanser
1 part yellow dock—Blood purifier, liver cleanser, kidney cleanser
½ part sarsaparilla—Binds with toxins
1 part elderberry—Removes pathogens
1 part hydrangea root—Breaks up calcification

Mix all parts thoroughly in blender. Make 500 mg capsules or quarter-teaspoon doses (1/2g). Dosage: two capsules two or three times daily. Take them for 1 -2 months.

How to rejuvenate your kidney, bladder?

With Whole Watermelon Juice out of the fruit and rind and that is the best! It even tastes good!

If you don't have a good juicer, put the whole watermelon in a blender with water, blend it and then filter the particles out with a cotton bag.

In the watermelon rind are 95% of the nutrition and you cannot get them when you eat the watermelon!

The whole watermelon juice will:

Cleanse our urogenital canal, kidneys and bladder, so it is very similar and close to cranberry juice.

Detox and cleanse our blood.

Stimulates our sex drive and is called the natural Viagra!

Contribute to a healthy prostate.

Has Tons of Pro-vitamin A, Potassium, Zinc (fights impotency), Lycopene (fights cancer).

The best source for L-Arginine & L-Citrulline that will open our blood vessels wider for more blood flow (good for sport and potency).

Is very alkaline in our body and so counteract against an acid body.

Drink 800ml/day in the morning, add 20ml apple cider and miracles will happen!

Best to drink before breakfast or before any meal.

In addition, eat every day one cucumber… it's so good for our heart, kidneys, body…

Or juice the cucumber…

How to kill the Parasites in our body?

Today I want to cover the best herbs for parasites.

A parasite is a microorganism like a worm or bacteria that basically lives off of your body but doesn't give you anything back.

Even though your friendly bacteria live off of your body, they are not parasites because they can actually do things for you, such as:

To help your digestion.
To kill harmful organism and bacteria.
Give your immune system protection.
Help make certain vitamins.
Help make antioxidants.
Help with your blood sugar.

How to find out that we have parasites in our body?

A few symptoms that can occur if someone has parasites:

Fatigue
Weight loss
Itchy private parts
Bloating
Nausea
Diarrhea

The best remedies for parasites:

1. Wormwood supplement
2. Black walnut hulls tincture

3. Clove supplements (the clove bought in the supermarket will not work!)
4. Garlic, good fresh big garlic cloves 3 times/day 1 clove
5. Apple vinegar, cider 3times/day 1 teaspoon

From Kroeger Herb you can buy the complete supplement (wormwood, clove and black walnut tincture, you take the recommend doses from each herb) for the parasites…
You can buy it from I-herbs…

When you do a parasite cleanse, you may want to do it for at least one month. You could even do it for six weeks before you stop taking it and see how you do. It's not a bad idea to do this, every six months when you have/had parasites.

If you're trying to get rid of a parasite, you should avoid certain foods, such as:

Sugar
Refined carbohydrates
Milk

Taking apple cider vinegar on a regular basis may also be beneficial to help kill off parasites.

Before you start with these herbs,
You start with detoxing of your liver with Milk Thistle for at least 2 weeks, or better for 4 to 6 weeks… Because the herbs in this list will detox your body and then you can become sick by the detoxing…

The other choice is to take Bile salt supplement for at least one day… But it is hard to buy and expensive… I know only Amazon and eBay…

Take 3 capsules of bile salt on an empty stomach, one in the morning, one in the early afternoon one before you go to bed.

And then start with

1. Wormwood supplement
2. Black walnut hulls tincture
3. Clove supplements (the clove bought in the supermarket will not work!)
4. Garlic good fresh big garlic cloves 3 times/day 1 clove
5. Apple vinegar cider 3times/day 1 teaspoon

Start with a minimum dose one of each for the day and increase the doses until you have reached the recommend level.

Do the detox for at least one month and not more than 6 weeks.
If you feel better repeat the parasite detox after a half year…

The Best Qigong

The Energy Pump

1. Every baby does this, and if the baby does this secret technique, they are experiencing a very high state of meditation!

2. Everybody can do this!

3. You can experience bliss, inner peace, and even more, but that is not all!

4. If you want to increase your ability to think, even if you are elderly, this is possible! Do you want to know this secret technique?

5. If you have problems with your bladder or urination problems, this secret technique will help.

6. The same goes for prostate problems/diseases.

7. I cured my back problems, including broken discs, and protruding discs that were pinching my nerves with this secret technique, my back got even better than it was before!

8. Men can control their orgasms. Women, would you like that?

9. Even more, you can enjoy sexual intercourse for as long as you want; believe me when I tell you that I even get stomach muscle cramps, so I have to keep changing the position.

10. Even better, you experience so much bliss that you lose your interest in the orgasms. Even better news is that multi orgasms for men are possible with this secret technique.

11. Your stamina during sex will increase along with your potency.

I will explain every point you need to exercise this technique until it works well for you, especially when you don't have experience in Qigong. For sure, bladder problems can be solved on the same day!

Males and females are different, do you agree? Ladies first! Females should squeeze their vagina and their anus, but should not squeeze the buttocks muscle.

Males should pull up their testicles, add some tension to their penis and squeeze their anus; they should not squeeze the buttocks muscle. You got it, is this easy? We call this energy pump!

Imagine that you are a baby who is sucking milk from the nipple of your mother's breast; when you are sucking milk, you assume that you are sucking the energy from your sex chakra upwards to the heart or even higher, while you maintain your energy pump. When you have sucked the energy, you should then breathe in; if you have breathed in enough air, then you need to breathe out, so you release the energy pump. Exactly as every baby does!! During the whole procedure, roll your tongue upwards and press the tip of your tongue against the top of the roof of your mouth.

We will support this by moving the palms of our hands upwards from the sex chakra to the head/crone chakra (See the Fulfilling Heart and the Fulfilling Bliss Qigong).

The same technique without moving your hands can be applied during intercourse, it is even better if also you repeat the name of God/ thank you / or another word that is meaningful to you.

Briefly, the problem for males is that during regular intercourse, men focus too much on the penis, so we need to lead the energy from our penis/testicles to our heart/crone chakra so that bliss occurs.

Apply the energy pump during meditation, this means 5 to 10 seconds, and also, repeat the name of God, or thank you, or another word that is meaningful to you. I count with the name of God. 5 times Krishna/Allah. Do this 50 to 100 times and then wait some time and then repeat as often as you like. You don't have to suck the energy upwards.

Better Thinking: You do the energy pump and suck the energy to the highest point of your head, this is the crone chakra. Do this 100 times a day (with the Fulfilling Heart and the Fulfilling Bliss you do that).

Bladder/ sexual stamina/ potency: energy pump, 5 seconds, repeating the name of God. do this 100 times.

The Fulfilling Heart

This is a simple great Qigong exercise for the heart. We experience bliss through the Energy Pump and moving the body. If we are agitated or have problems, this Fulfilling Heart Method will help a lot. See and download my video: https://goo.gl/LuNwP9 (https://s3-ap-southeast-1.amazonaws.com/rudizimmerer/video/The+fulfilling+Heart.mp4)

Never exercise with straight knees or straight arms. The joints should be loose, the knee is bent so that the knee is actually above the foot, half way to the tip of the toes. This is recommended to do always, never stand with straight knees. Otherwise the energy can't flow.

Do the Fulfilling Heart Qigong between 24 to 30 cycles for every minute and as long as you like.

During the whole procedure, roll your tongue upwards and press the tip of your tongue against the top of the roof of your mouth.

I assume that you have learned the Energy Pump already.

We will improve the Energy Pump with body movements.

1. You breathe in, your body should be bent a little forward, arms loose at your side, palms directed forward, body weight forward. Do energy pump. Swing the body upwards so that the spine becomes straight and with this movement, swing the arms forwards until they are nearly above the head with the palms facing forward, raise up the heel at the end. Imagine that you are throwing your loose arms with your body movements upwards.

2. You breathe out, release the Energy Pump, swing your body downward, swing your arms downward and turn the palms

downward; put your body weight backward and drop the heel on the ground.

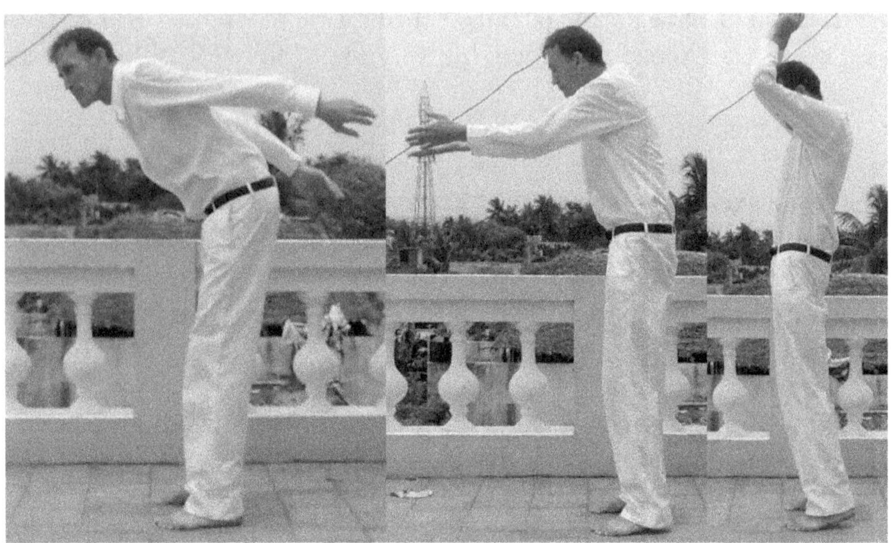

In the first two pictures we see the forward movement with palms facing forward while breathing in, and the third picture we can see that the palms are turned downward, heels lifted up, and you should breathe out.

The Fulfilling Bliss

I have used the Fulfilling Bliss method every day for over ten years. If I feel agitated or can't sleep this Qigong exercise really helps. The Fulfilling Bliss method is a great moving meditation that gives us so many benefits: See and download my video: https://goo.gl/RrcXqg (https://s3-ap-southeast-1.amazonaws.com/rudizimmerer/video/The+Fulfilling+Bliss.mp4)

1. We experience bliss

2. We heal our spine and our body

3. We transform negative feelings to bliss

4. We get peace in our mind and serenity

5. We learn to send energy out of our hands and get eventual healing hands

6. For a good deep sound sleep

7. We improve our thinking

8. We improve our bladder and sexual stamina

9. Our energy is circulating from the sexual organ through the spine until the crone chakra and over the mouth through our heart, stomach, navel chakra back to the sexual organ. This will cure many diseases and strengthen our immune system. This energy circulation is the same as from the Immortal Qigong and called Macro Cosmos by Mantak Chia.

It is quite a challenge to learn in the beginning because today our movements are not so round and elastic. So it is much easier to learn if we had learned first the Fulfilling Heart Qigong.

During the whole procedure, roll your tongue upwards and press the tip of your tongue against the top of the roof of your mouth.

We use the Energy Pump again to bring our energy upward when we breathe in and downward when we breathe out.

We use three different movements, body, arms/hands, and feet. These movements are synchronized to our breathing. Within 1 minute we have 24 to 30 cycles of breathing/ movements/ energy pump. We use the natural speed of our body, not too fast and not too slow. We make the Fulfilling Bliss 10 to 30 minutes so that it works. I do this exercise 5 times a day.

We have eight different arm/hand movements, so the body and foot movement remain the same.

If we breathe out, we move the arms with the hands forward from our body away and the body/back/weight we move backward, so from the hands away. In the end position our body is bent forward like a bow and the arms are straight, only a little bit bent so that the energy can flow.

If we breathe in, we pull the arms back to the body and the body/weight we move forward. In the end position, our body is bent backward like a bow.

The heels are going upward if we start to inhale, and are going downwards if we change from inhaling to exhaling. At the pivot point from exhaling to inhaling, our heel is touching the ground. And when we start to breathe out, our heels are already raised upward.

We always use the shortest way to reach the end position of our hands. The end position is where we change from exhaling to inhaling.

We learn eight different end positions of the hands.

Now the fine tuning:

We send energy with our eyes and hands out if we breathe out. The fingers are straight, but still loose and the eyes are looking sharp. When we breathe in, we pull the energy out of the ground and navel chakra upwards to our crone chakra. This time we look inwards, with a soft look, and the finger joints are softly bent inside as though we want to scratch something.

We have eight different hand positions, and the last sequence, you bow your body forward much more than the other sequences.

Now I will describe the various hand positions for the different end positions from the eight sequences:

1. Both palms of your hands are facing each other, the distance is 1 to 2 times of your head width, 5 to 10 inches in front of your face.

2. Both palms of your hands are facing upwards, the distance is 1 to 2 times of your head width, 5 to 10 inches in front of your face.

3. Both palms of your hands are facing each other, the distance is 1 to 1.5 times of your hips width, height is the navel, the elbow should be bent 100^0 to $135^0.$

4. Both palms of your hands are facing downwards, the distance is 1 to 1.5 times of your hips width, height is the navel, the elbow should be bent 100^0 to 135^0.

5. Both palms of your hands are facing downwards, the distance is 1 to 1.5 times of your hips width, height is the navel, the elbow should be bent 100^0 to 135^0. This time your hands move in addition to sequence 4 in a circle. You start outwards (both

hands have here 2 times hips width distance from each other) at the pivot point. Then you circle the hands nearer to each other so that they have only 1/2 to 1-time hip width distance from each other. Then again you circle them outside until they have 1 to 1.5 times the hip width.

6. Both palms of your hands are facing upwards, the distance is 1 to 1.5 times of your hips width, height is the navel, the elbow should be bent at 100^0 to 135^0.

7. Both palms of your hands are facing upwards, the distance is 1 to 1.5 times of your hips width, height is one hand width under the navel, the elbow should be bent at 100^0 to 135^0.

Both palms of your hands are facing each other, the distance is 1 to 1.5 times of your hips width, height is under the knees, this means you bow down your body, the elbow should be bent 100^0 to 135^0.

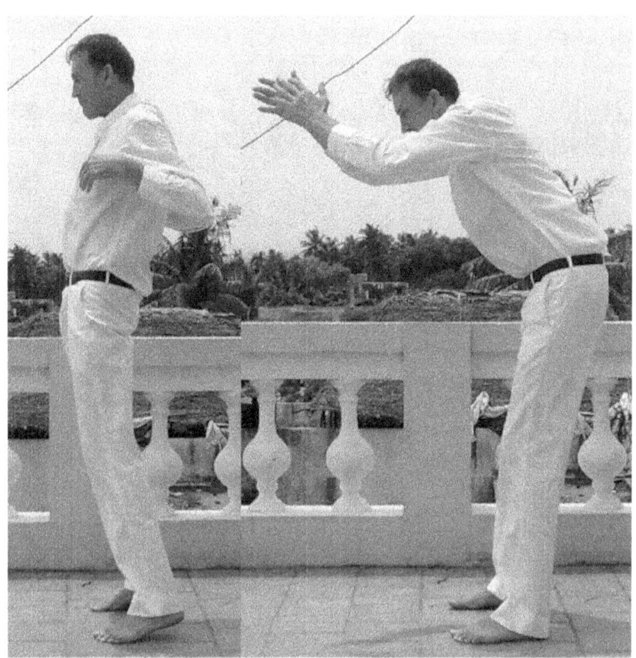

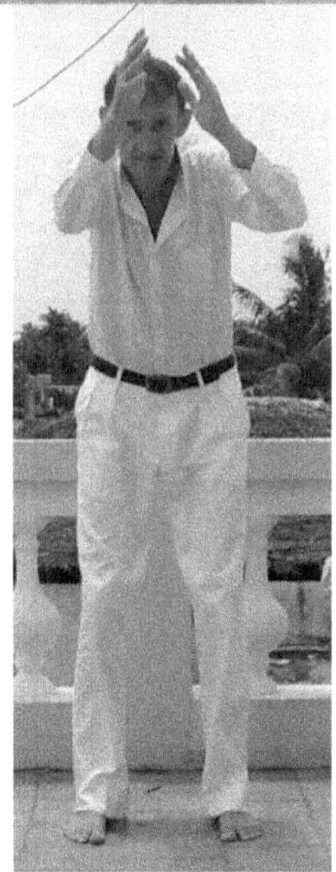

These are the pictures from Sequence 1

In picture 1: I go backwards with my body and arms, the heels are raised up, and my body has a backward bow with my finger joints bent inside.

In pictures 2 and 3: I go forwards with my body and arms, the heels are touching the ground, my body has a forward bow and fingers are straight.

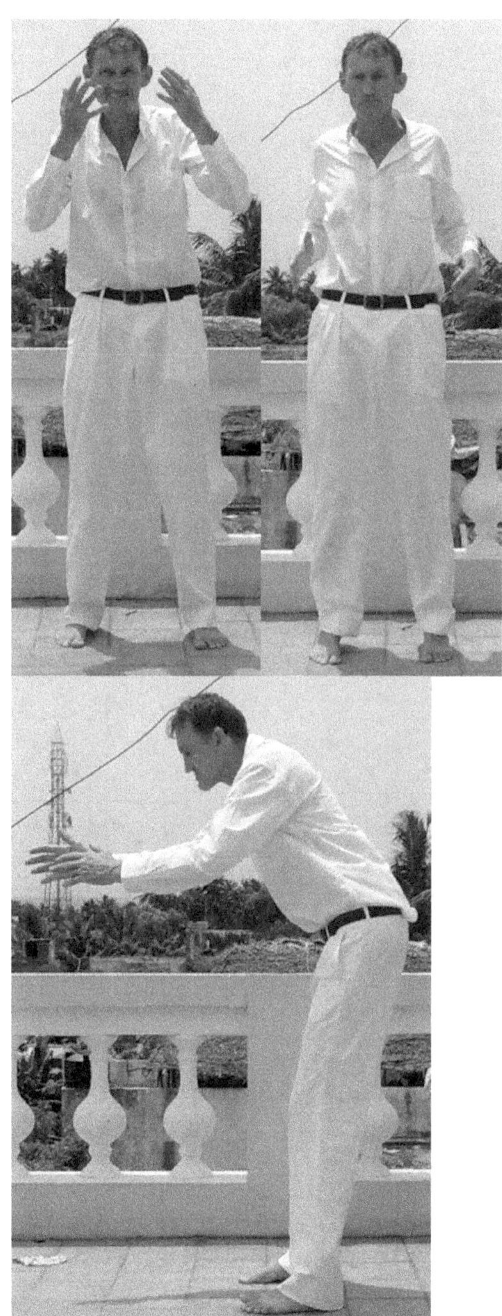

Picture 1: Sequence2, forward movement

Picture 2: Sequence3 backward movement

Picture 3: Sequence4 forward movement.

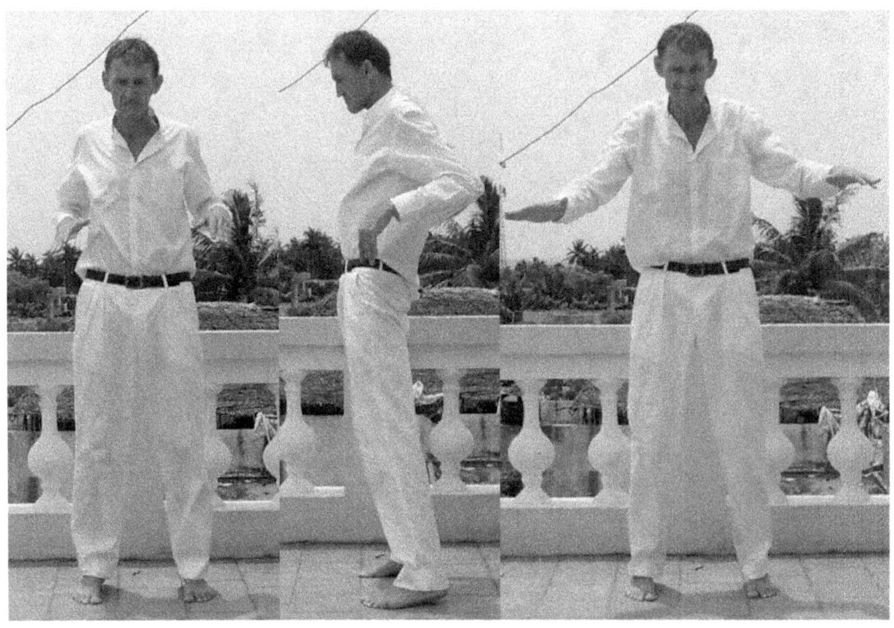

Picture 1: Sequence4 forward movement.

Picture 2: Sequence4 backward movement

Picture 3: Sequence5 forward movement.

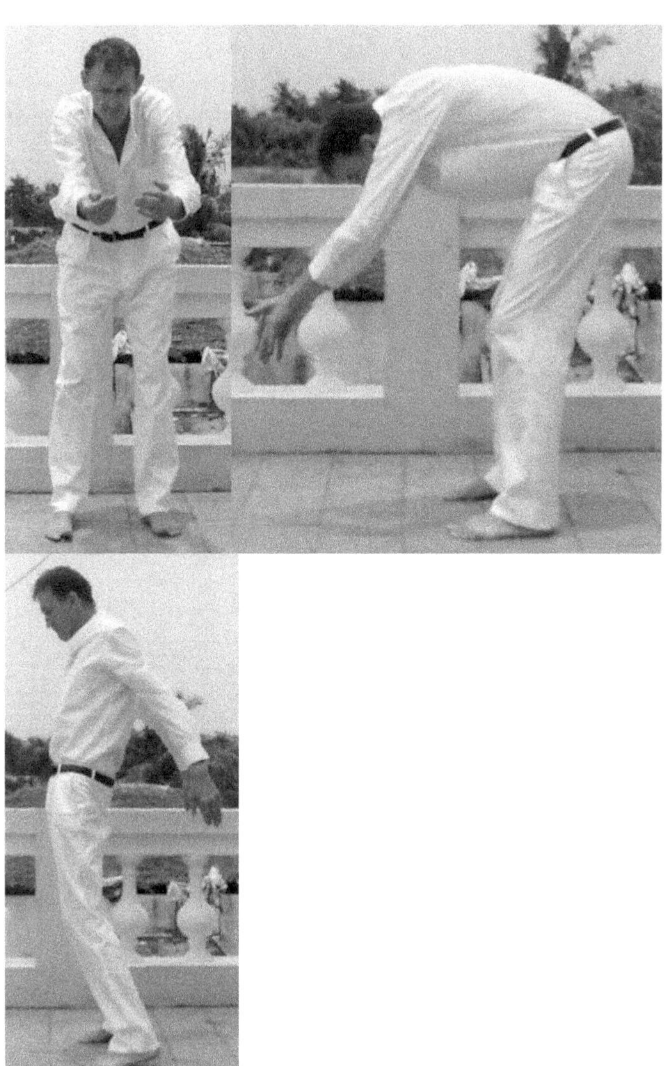

Picture 1: Sequence7 backward movement.

Picture 2: Sequence8 forward movement

Picture 3: Sequence8 forward movement.

If we have mastered the Fulfilling Bliss and the Immortal Qigong we can use the Golden Pill for the Fulfilling Bliss. We project the Golden Pill on the Mingmen and pulling it upwards. If we have mastered that, then we repeat silently "Who Ohm" and a name of God that resonant with the higher Chakras.

The Tao 5 Elements to release negative feelings and to heal.

With these exercises, we can release our suppressed negative feelings: anger, worry, sadness, impatience, stress, and fear. We can also heal our organs with the Five Elements. See my Video: https://youtu.be/sSkamsxM46U

I have tried out more than 100 Qigong exercises, and honestly, most of them don't have many benefits. I have chosen from different teachers the most effective techniques for the Five Elements. I don't care about tradition, I only care about results. At first, we make the 5 healing sounds of the 5 Elements loud, after some months we can make them also remote. See and download my video: https://goo.gl/N5PmB1 (https://s3-ap-southeast-1.amazonaws.com/rudizimmerer/video/The+Tao+5+Elements.mp4)

Sit down on a chair and close your eyes for all 5 elements.

Anger

If we get angry quite fast, then our anger level is too high. Anger is related to the liver or to the Wood element. I have chosen here the inner organ massage, tapping combined with the sound of 'Sh.' - The virtue of the liver is compassion. So we have to transform our anger into compassion. And it works. On the right side of our body, under the rib cage is the liver. We approach the rib cage from the belly and then grip with both hands under our rib cage as deeply as possible. Start to massage the liver under the rib cage and make the sound 'Sh'. After some time we alter the procedure, then tap this area on the ribs with one hand, lay the other hand below the navel and continuously make the 'Sh' sound. We can now feel our anger, so let it go. This procedure we do for 3- 5 minutes. At the end, we place both hands above our liver and feel thankful for our liver and imagine that a green light is entering our liver.

Worry

If we have too much worry, then I have chosen the inner organ massage again and tapping for the spleen, combined with the sound of 'Hu' (English word sound is "Who") or the Earth Element. The virtues of the spleen are fairness and openness. On the left side under the rib cage is the spleen. We approach the rib cage from the belly and then grip with both hands under our rib cage as deeply as possible. Start to massage the spleen under the rib cage while making the sound 'Hu'. After some time we alter the procedure then tap this area with one hand on the ribs and the other below the navel, while continuously making the 'Hu' sound. We can now feel our worry, so let it go. This procedure we do for 3- 5 minutes. At the end, we put both hands above our spleen and feel thankful for our spleen and imagine that a yellow light is entering our spleen.

Sadness and Grief

For Sadness and Grief is the lung or metal element. The sound for this is a sharp 'S' (like Song). I have chosen the tapping. The virtues of the lungs are courage and rightness, so we have to transform our sadness and grief to courage and rightness. We tap our rib cage from both sides with both fists. We can alter, if we tap with one hand the rib cage, and lay the other hand below our navel (lower dantien - below the navel). We tap, making the sound 'S' (loud or mute) and feel our sadness and grief, now let go of them. Do this procedure for 3 to 5 minutes. At the end, we place both hands above our lungs and feel thankful for them while imagining that white light is entering our lungs.

Stress and Impatience

For Stress (fear combined with anger for a particular outcome) and impatience, is the heart or Fire element, the sound is 'Haw.' The virtue of the heart is love. So we have to transform our stress and impatience to love. Here I have chosen the healing sound exercise. We start to breathe in and spread our arms to the left and right side and then raise them up with the palms upward in a big circle above the head. They should touch each other with the finger tips, (now the palms are downward, because of the circle we have made). Move them down to you head; then we join them and interlace them; turn the palms upwards, and straighten them upwards, so the left hand is pulling the right upwards, so that the body moves a little bit to the right side. We breathe out and make the sound 'Haw'. With the sound, we release our stress and impatience. When we have exhaled all the air, we push our hands further upwards so that they separate, and again in a big circle we move the arms downward and lay them on our lap. Rest for one inhale and exhale, and repeat this procedure for 3 to 5 minutes. At the end, we place both hands above our heart and feel thankful for our heart. Now we imagine that a red light is entering our heart. See the pictures beneath for help with these steps.

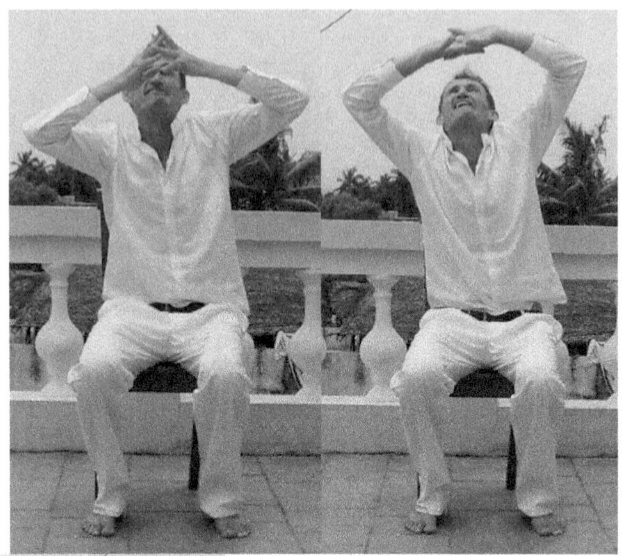

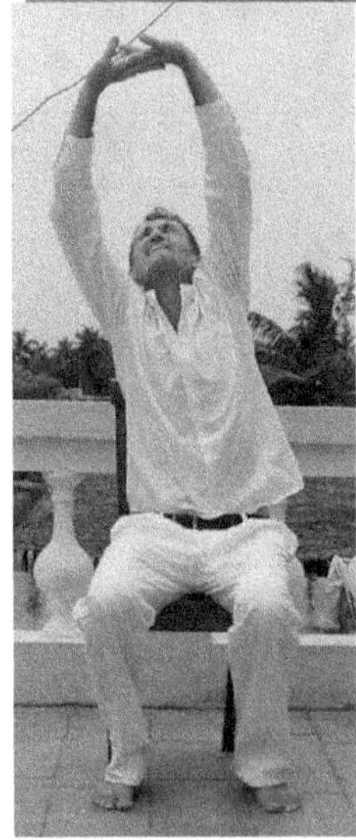

Deep Fear

For deep fear is the kidneys and element water. The sound is 'Cho.' The virtues of the kidneys are calmness and gentleness. We have to transform our deep fear to calmness and gentleness. I have chosen the healing sound exercise with rubbing our kidneys when we have bowed our back forward and do the sound " Cho." We sit on a chair, feet on the ground, raise up the heels so that we give more power on our kidney reflexology points under the feet. We bow forward that our head is nearly touching our knees. We breathe deep in and out from our belly. We make the sound 'Cho' and when we feel our fear, we let go of it. We clap our hands rub the palms against each other until they are warm. We put both hands on the area of our kidneys and rub the area of our kidneys. We keep making the sound "Cho" and to rub the kidneys in the described position for 3 to 5 minutes. When the rubbing of the kidneys is too exhausting, rest for a while the hands on the kidneys and then continue. In the end, we feel thankful for them. We imagine that blue light is entering our kidneys. See the pictures beneath for help with these steps.

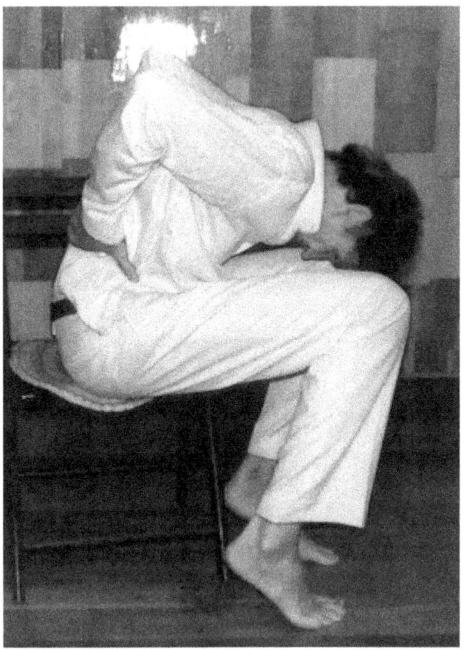

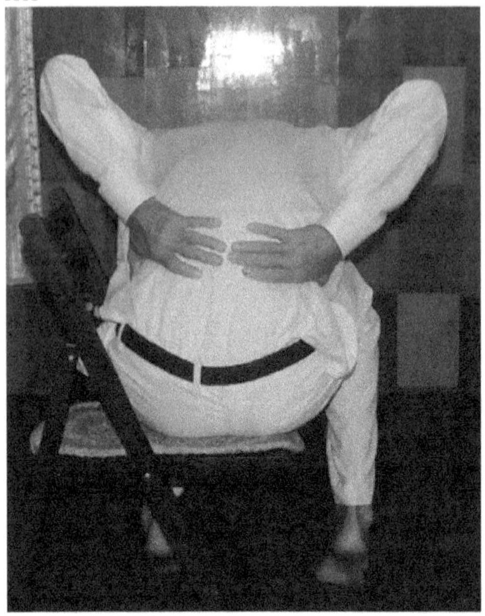

The best Therapy - EFT

Emotion Freedom Techniques

Emotional Freedom Techniques (EFT) is based on Chinese acupuncture. The theory is that we have energy blockages in our body caused by suppressed feelings. EFT is a combination of tapping certain acupuncture points with addressing the suppressed feelings. When every other therapy failed, EFT has worked. This became true for the Vietnam veterans who had such deep traumas they were suffering and no therapy could help them. EFT did.

EFT is easy to learn and requires five minutes for suppressed negative feelings, and ten to thirty minutes for traumas. Imagine wanting to meditate when you are troubled by negative thoughts. Negative thoughts are caused by negative feelings, and EFT helps you get free from them within minutes.

Description of EFT

EFT is simple to apply (There are very many websites for EFT, for instance http://www.eftuniverse.com/).

First, we investigate our problem with all of our feelings. Then we investigate which kind of feelings are attached to our problem, and which context the feelings are to our problem. For instance, we are angry because we lost money on the stock market.

If that's the case, I am angry about losing money, and I am angry because I did not keep my trading rules. I am angry that the price of the stock went down. I am angry because big traders had manipulated this price and I am angry because I estimated wrong. I am fearful to lose money again with the next trade. I am so anxious that I never will trade again. I am afraid to become rich and successful. I am afraid to have more money than my family, and I am afraid that I am smarter than other people, etc. So we have to apply for every feeling EFT.

We are not embarrassed to look at every feeling of our problem, because if we do not find all the connected feelings from our problem, EFT is not working. Then for every feeling (in this example are ten emotions), we estimate the strength of this feeling on a scale between one and ten. A ten is the strongest feeling, and a one is the lowest. We then explore this feeling/problem but not too deep. Crying is okay but try not to get too intensive. We feel our body. If the feeling does not coming up by itself, then we act like an actor and imagine the feeling in a hypothetical situation until we feel this emotion. Or, we postpone the EFT.

Afterward, we articulate this specific feeling/problem with this sentence: Even though I have this . . . (fear of losing money, headache, craving for alcohol, war memory, nightmares, headache, insomnia . . .) (address only one feeling), I deeply love and completely accept myself (or use a similar sentence).

At the same time, we rub our **WP** Sore point or hit our **KP** Karate point (you will find it later in my book) with our index and middle finger seven to ten times. We repeat this three times.

Then we speak out our feelings/problems, for what we like to make EFT and feel it.

Articulate: Fear of losing money, at the same time we tap our skull with the palm of our hand seven times and then we tap with our index and middle finger every EFT point (see later).

WP sore point: We have two sore points that are located on the chest. If you draw a line between the breast nipple and the U-shape notch of your sternum, then one-quarter to one-third from the nipple is a point (1-inch radius) that aches when you press it. This is the sore point.

K   skull tap with the palm of your hand

AB   beginning of the eyebrow

SA   side of the eye

UA   under the eye

UN   under the nose

KI   chin: midway between the point of the chin and the bottom of the lower lip

SB   beginning of the collarbone: one thumb width under and outside of collarbone

UA   under the arm and at the height of the breast nipple - tap with fists

DA   side of the thumb, outside of hand, at a point even with the base of the thumbnail

ZF   index finger side, facing thumb at a point even with the base of nail,

MF   middle finger side index finger, facing index finger, at a point even with the base of nail

KF pinky finger side, facing ring finger, at a point even with the base of nail,

KP karate chop edge of hand, one-third-length of karate edge from pinky finger

And then comes the 9 Gamut procedures

Here you tap always on the GM Gamut-point (between the knuckles at the base of the ring finger and the pinky finger, one thumb width under the knuckles)

1. Eyes closed

2. Eyes open

3. Eyes down and right

4. Eyes down and left

5. Roll eyes in a circle (clockwise): imagine your nose is the center of the clock and you're trying to see all numbers

6. Roll eyes counter-clockwise in reverse direction

7. Hum a song for 2 seconds (Happy Birthday for example)

8. Count rapidly from 1 to 5

9. Hum for 2 seconds again

After one lap, we estimate on our scale how strong our feeling/problem is. If we are above 2, then we make the next lap until we are below 2. For the next laps, we add the word still.

Even though I still have fear . . .

If you are in public and are embarrassed to do EFT, then do the EFT in your mind by imaging the whole procedure.

Please avoid negative sentences if possible. Omit the words 'no' and 'not'.

Example: I am jealous.

Aspects can be anger, fear that our partner will leave us, fear that we are not good enough, and fear that our perception is right and jealous.

First aspect: Even though I am (still) angry that Jane sleeps with another man, I love and accept me as I am. (We do not care if it is true or not true; the feeling is important.)

Tapping with: (still) angry that Jane.

Second aspect: Even though I am (still) afraid that Jane will leave me, I love and accept me as I am. I will find a new, cuter, more beautiful darling.

Tapping with: (still) afraid that Jane will leave me.

Third aspect: Even though I am (still) afraid that her new darling is better than me, I love and accept me as I am. And I know that I am the better one.

Tapping with: (still) afraid that her new darling is better than me.

Forth aspect: Even though I am (still) afraid that Jane is with another man, I love and accept me as I am.

Tapping with: (still) afraid Jane is with another man.

Fifth aspect: Even though I am (still) jealous about Jane's darling, I love and accept me as I am. I know I will find a better, cuter, and more beautiful darling.

Taping with: (still) jealous about Jane's darling.

We all get many things in our life on a daily basis that we cannot emotionally digest, so we suppress our negative emotion. If we apply EFT every day, we can stay open, and we will transform our entire lives to a more happy and relaxed one.

If we compare ourselves with young children--how open and spontaneous they are--then we understand why EFT is so necessary for us.

Emotional cleaning with EFT

We list all our struggles and traumas from our entire life, and then we apply EFT for all of them. The reasons for such cleaning are that the suppressed feelings of struggles and traumas can cause severe diseases or are a hindrance to be open and happy now.

If we cannot feel the traumas or struggles anymore, the suppressed feelings are still inside us. Then we make some more rounds up to ten times; do not be lazy. Give yourself time for this emotional cleaning, One to five months should be enough.

My Own EFT

Gary Craig, the founder of EFT, had inspired his students to create their own EFT in order to get it better done. I took all the EFT points from the basic course, and added three major acupuncture points to it.

Gary tried to use less EFT points in order to make it faster work; I have done the opposite, because I have more understanding from acupuncture than him. For me, my EFT is more effective and even faster than his version, because we need fewer laps.

Both versions work best if you go through the sequence of the EFT points. I added **SP** stress point, **WU** anger point, the **Si4** major acupuncture point, and the **TAT** basic position. The other EFT points are part of the basic courses like **AP** anxiety point, **UP** under-pulse point, **WA** wade point, **NAA** neck skull back edge point, and **NAM** neck skull back middle point.

K　skull tap with the palm of hand

AB　beginning of eyebrow

SA　side of the eye

UA　under the eye

UN　under nose

KI　chin: midway between the point of chin and the bottom of lower lip

SP　stress point in the cave behind earlobe; rub with index finger

SB　beginning of collarbone: one thumb width under and outside collarbone

UA　under the arm and in the height of breast nipple tapping with fists

Tap both hands against each other on the points **UP, AP, and KP**

UP　under pulse point: three thumbs wide behind base of hand, palm side

AP   anxiety point: end of the edge of hand (karate) on the knuckle

KP   karate-chop edge of hand: one-third length of karate-chop edge from pinky finger

DA   thumb side of thumb, outside of hand, at a point even with the base of thumbnail

SI4 major acupuncture point: hand outside, flesh between index finger and thumb

ZF   index finger: side index finger, facing thumb, at a point even with the base of nail,

MF   middle finger: side index finger, facing index finger, at a point even with the base of nail,

KF   pinky finger: side pinky finger, facing ring finger, at a point even with the base of nail,

GM Gamut-point (between the knuckles at the base of the ring finger and the pinky finger, one thumb width under the knuckles)

WA wade point: one hand width above foot knuckle; tap with both palms inside and outside

WU anger point: one thumb width behind and between base of big toe and next toe

Middle line of body front side; tap with both fists from the pubic bone up to the neck.

TAT position with thumb and ring finger: press nose bone and inside edge of eye caves; with middle finger press the third eye (where Hindus paint the red point)

TAT+ NAA neck skull back edge point is base of skull, backside, the edge, first left; tap with fist.

TAT+ NAM   neck skull back middle point is base of skull, back side, the middle; tap with fist.

TAT+ NAA   neck skull back edge point is base of skull, backside, the edge, and right; tap with fist.

Tap the finger points only on one side, then on the other side. Or, tap with the left and the right hand finger against each other.

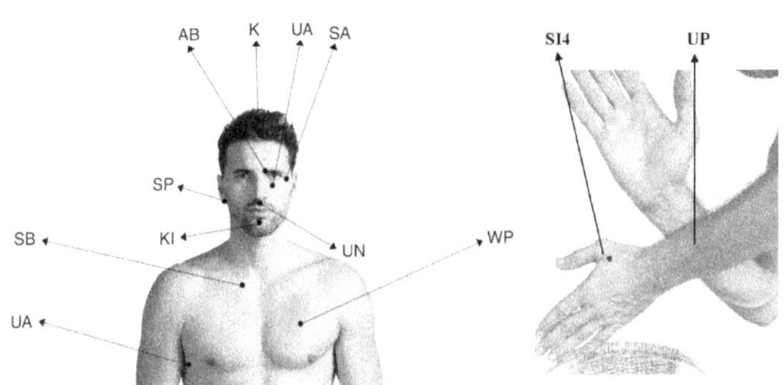

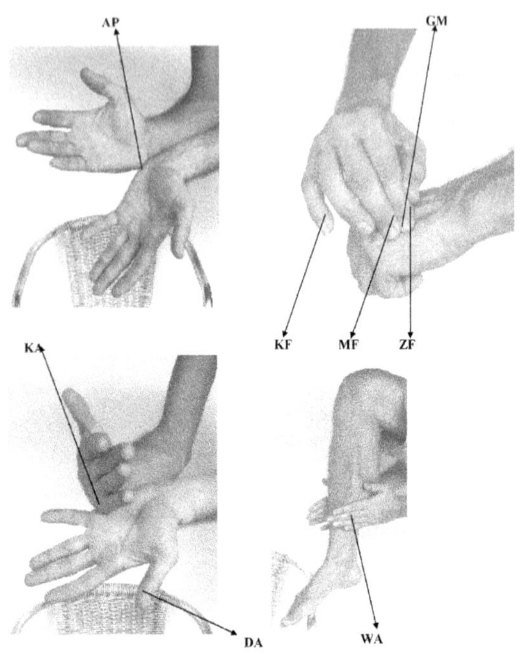

AP
GM
KF
MF
ZF
KA
DA
WA

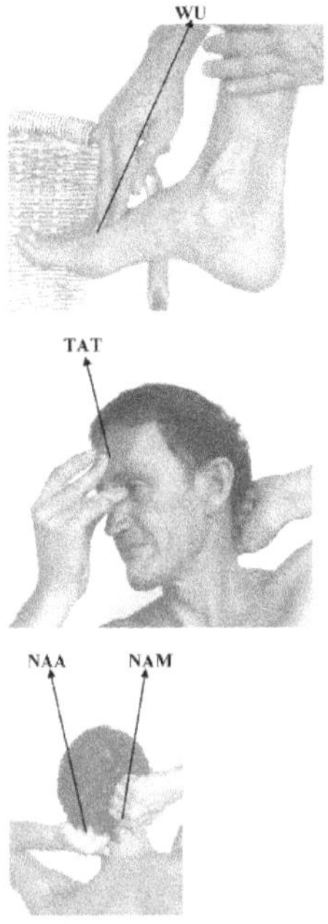

We do my EFT the same way like the version of Billy Craig, without the 9 Gamut procedures.

After we do all laps from my EFT, we do eye movements. Move your thumb from left to right and then back to left in front of your eyes, about fifteen to twenty inches away. Follow the thumb with your eyes in a horizontal middle line; do this 3 times. Then move the thumb in a diagonal line, from down left to up right and back; follow the thumb with your eyes: 3 times. Then move the thumb in a diagonal line, from down right to up left and then back; follow the thumb with your eyes: 3 times. Do not move the head. The whole procedure takes about two minutes.

Heal yourself and stay healthy!

The Best Alternative Drugs/Herbs

Alternative medications: **Colloidal silver** doses 15ppm till 50ppm. Typical doses are for bacterial infection 2-3 times, 1Table-spoonful every day for 7 to 14 days. (Side effects begin with 400l/year). You can produce it by yourself, but then you will harm the pharmacy. It will not kill the bacteria in the bowels.

Bladder inflammation take **cranberries**… Get dried cranberries. Don't buy the cranberry juice because the cranberry juice is acid. Put 70g dried cranberries in warm water; blend them in a blender; wait for 10 minutes and blend them again… And then drink 2 times per day this Cranberry juice for 14 days.

Disinfection: **Tea tree oil** You can apply directly on the infected wound.
Disinfection: **Turmeric - powder**, an excellent anti-inflammation for wounds, also suitable for bowels inflammation/ulcer when you eat it.

For fungus in the ear or vagina: **Garlic oil** (put garlic in oil to infuse for one day) and apply 5 times a day for one week.

Thyme for the lungs, drink it with ginger and lemon or steam bath.

Flaxseed as Omega alpha 3 oil for the brain, nerves, and eyes. Don't buy the supplement because the digest system can't assimilate the Omega alpha 3 oil out of the supplement. Get a blender; put 3 to 4 table-spoon flaxseed in a blender; grind it well; add enough water, blend it again; wait at least for 10 minutes and eat it.

Gelatin for joints and disc growth.

Fish collagen capsules (3capsules/day) or 10g gelatin/day soaked in water, for growing our joints with exercises for 3 to 5 month. Also, Dr. John Bergman recommends this.

The best alternative Remedies

Allergy healing with Bioresonance and much more

We had a huge problem with the daughter X of our great herbalist…

His daughter X had so much water in her lungs that she could not leave the bed and the water had to be removed by surgery…

What to do?

I assumed that the cause is/was allergy…

And for allergy works at best Bioresonance Therapy *, developed by German science…
The Bioresonance therapy is using a device that normalize our organ and body frequencies.
Every organ has a specific frequency and if the organ is not functioning well his frequency becomes unhealthy…

The international results are 80 to 90% to cure Allergy with Bioresonance!!!!!

But there are only three clinics in Thailand who are doing the Bioresonance Therapy…

I said to our old partial retired Herbal Doctor, you cannot lose anything… Go to Hua Hin and try this cure, if you have questions, the doctor of the clinic is even a Professor of TCM.

Our herbal doctor went there… because otherwise his daughter would have never any chance to leave the bed…

Bingo!!!! Yes, the Bioresonance therapy works also for X… After 4month laying in the bed, she starts now to walk and that only after 2 treatments!!!

I got this tip from the business Mogul Hugh Hilton (interview with J.T. Fox)…. Hugh Hilton had a severe accident and after the accident, his Adrenaline increases, so high that his blood pressure and heart beat could kill him… And he could not bring it down without taking very many drugs.

What to do, he heard from Bioresonance therapy, after one session, he felt like to be young again and the Adrenaline level was normal. Now, he is doing every second week Bioresonance therapy to feel young again…

There are no international studies to improve other diseases for instance like cancer with Bioresonance… Still, it can work…

There exists only one firm (Bicom) who are producing these Bioresonance devices… all the other Bioresonance devices are fake!!!
It was very difficult and expensive to get a Bicom device, because I am not a doctor, even I have studied medicine as an engineer… (It fits perfectly to my background, Western medicine and Chinese healing). Now I am waiting to get the Bicom 2000 plus, second hand, …

With this device you can make also Electrical Acupuncture after Voll (German science) (EAV) to analyze and cure diseases…
This I am learning right now…

Selenium for a stronger immune system

After many years the science found the benefits of Selenium for our body.
Selenium will:

Strengthen your immunity.
Benefit our heart.
Lowering blood pressure.
Powerful antioxidant.
Helps the intestines absorb nutrients.
Prevents muscle cramping.
Normalize our hormone levels.
Strengthening bones.
Prevents goiters and improves blood circulation!

Most of all people have a deficit of Selenium, like me, and so we should add more.
Our daily source should at least be 55mg.

And there is one nut, that has 40 times more selenium than any other natural source of selenium.

1 Brazil nut has 60 - 90mg Selenium.
We need only to consume 2 - 3 Brazil nuts.
The best is to grind the Brazil nut and soak it in water… I add it to my Flaxseed (omega alpha oil source), grind it …
Don't eat too much Brazil nuts, not more than 5 because it has too much calories…
If you eat the Brazil nut, you have to chew it very much to get the benefits!

The health benefit of Brazil nut are:
A great source of vitamins such as vitamin B-complex.

It is also packed with minerals, Manganese, Selenium, Potassium, Calcium, Iron. Phosphorus and Zinc.
It is packed with anti-aging and immune-enhancing substances.
It is also rich in vitamin E and vitamin C.
Contain 14% protein

Does a Stem cell cure help?

Sure, it helps a lot to make big money.
Such miracle cures for reversing aging have existed for 1000 years and never have worked out…

When we age then our cells will get replaced more and more by cells that are not identical and so not functioning so well… That causes a damage in our organs…

The stem cells from different organs are the most important cells that can produce far more cells than other cells… If we reduce the number of stem cells, we reduce the cell growing and we increase the damage of cells…

If we grow older, our stem cells are reduced…

Honestly, do you think that this can be the major reason to get ill or to die?
For sure not!

All the life-threatening diseases can have also a young person, without a problem in his number of his stem cells.

A hospital doctor told me, that even very old people can have healthier and better functioning organs than a young person…

Certainly, reduced populations of our existing stem cells are not likely to be helpful to our tissues as we live over the years and decades.

We can increase naturally the number of stem cells… This I will explain later!

The fact that our stem cell numbers tend to decrease with age does not necessarily mean that stem cell treatments for aging make any sense. In fact, there are a lot of problems with the idea of infusions of stem cells to fight aging. First, most clinics selling this idea simply infuse fat (or amniotic) stem cells into the bloodstream, collect their thousands of dollars from customers, and then wave a magic wand or something.

There's good evidence that those fat stem cells injected into the bloodstream mostly are gone with hours or days, certainly within weeks. They are filtered out in the lungs (one reason for worrying about pulmonary emboli or blood clots in the lungs as a side effect) or elsewhere. Many probably die from the shock of entering the bloodstream or are killed by immune cells. In short, there's a very limited window of time that such cells could do anything helpful and the idea that during that window they could permanently help counteract aging seems like a snowball's chance in hell. Maybe bone marrow cells would have a relatively better chance.

And the bone marrow cells, we can increase with Iron Shirt III Qigong.

When we eat fermented vegetables every day, we increase our stem cells up to 4 times it depends on the organ.
I love my self-made Kimchi (Korean fermented vegetables), it is so healthy and taste so well. I don't care for the Stem cells.

With Qigong we increase the stem cells… That is the reason why these Qigong masters are living so long!

Now, Master Mantak Chia is offering Stem cell Qigong…
This Qigong was called before Iron Shirt II and III… Iron Shirt II and III and are very good, but Stem Cell Qigong sounds much better?

I make my Iron Shirt II combined with Iron Shirt III (I call it different in my book, because the name Iron Shirt sounds so bad) even before I knew that it produces more Stem Cells…

How to kill every virus, bacteria?

without using any medicaments…?

We can kill with Microamperes (0.1mA) every parasites, virus, and bacteria… in the blood…
And this works even with Aids…

Since nearly a hundred years, many Scientists like Rife, Dr. Bob Becker, Clark, and many German Scientists have proofed that micro amperes kill every virus…

He was using only 50 to 100 microamperes, 50 millionths of an ampere were all it needed, and it later turned out to neutralize or eliminate every parasite, every fungus, every germ, every bacteria, every virus in the blood [in the laboratory]. And it had no side effects, no adverse effect on the blood cells. We know what's happening now … my doctorate was in physics, a D.Sc. But here was probably the most important thing I'd seen in my lifetime, so I developed units.-Dr. Bob Beck Protocol. See link at the end.

If we apply and I have done so, for 2 hours every day for 6 weeks this microampere on the pulse of our hand wrist.

1.) the parasites, Virus, bacteria get killed in our blood….
2.) our body get detoxed
3.) accelerates overall healing…

Dr. Bob Becker designed a Zapper that creates these microamperes and even can produce Colloidal Silver (that also kills unhealthy bacteria), and he has given for free his design of this device… I have also built his Zapper… (you can get it from Sota, link at the end).

Never the less, still in our Lymph system and in our bone caves are the parasites…
And for that, we use an Electro-Magnetic Pulser that I own too (bought it from Sota)…

Still, if we kill all of our bacteria, we also kill our healthy bacteria… What to do??????

Eat probiotic as fermented vegetables 3 times a day when you use this Zapper or Electro-Magnetic Pulser… That is crucial; otherwise, your immune system is getting weak!

https://www.bobbeck.com

https://www.sota.com

https://www.bobbeck.com/pdfs/microcurrent-therapy.pdf

https://www.naturalhealthproductions.com/pdf/electricity-for-health-booklet.pdf

https://www.youtube.com/watch?v=1jXi3sc42nQ

How to cure a root Channel inflammation?

The root channel inflammation treatment from the dentists has the disadvantage that it kills the tooth and that the dead tooth in your mouth will attract harmful bacteria that can cause diseases.

For the root channel inflammation, the Indian dentists give you Antibiotics for 14 days; - most of the inflammation will be cured.

How is it if we substitute the antibiotic with Colloidal silver? Colloidal silver has nearly no side effects when we do not take more than 400 l a year. We need to take a spoon full of colloidal silver twice a day. My body is allergic to Antibiotics, and colloidal silver works for me. Colloidal silver works not for everybody, try it out for 3 days for some inflammations... If the colloidal silver works for you, then you can substitute it for Antibiotic.

For all inflammation, it is the best to take for at least 10 days the antibiotics or colloidal silver, to make sure the inflammation will not come back. My friends, who had studied medicine, told me that. Still, the doctors give us only 4 days Antibiotics so that we come back after 3 months.

The antibiotic kills all healthy bacteria in the guts and weakens so our immune system. After the antibiotic treatment, we eat everyday fermented vegetables, kefir, or take probiotic for 10 days to build up healthy bacteria in the guts. When we have healthy bacteria in the intestines, our body produces 4 times more stem cells! The best is to eat every day fermented vegetables or kefir.

How to prevent root channel inflammation?

1. If we feel pain when we are biting.

2. If we hit with a piece of steel (spoon) against the aching tooth and
    feel pain.
3. Tooth inflammation is caused by too much stress, told me a dentist
    working in the emergency service at the hospital. Get rid of
    stress!

These symptoms indicate us that we have a beginning of a root
channel inflammation…

We put 2 or 3 cloves in our mouth, chew them a little bit and let them
in the mouth for hours. Also, we chew ginger. We let both in our
mouth for hours. Slowly it will improve…

For people who have healing hands (Reiki) place a hand over your
mouth when you sleep. To make it even better use the healing sounds
"ee" "joe." You can make this sound loud or in silence.

I make the colloidal silver by myself with pure silver wire, distillate
water and 30V.

How to heal our Ears?

I used to have chronicle ear inflammation.
In the Past the ENT doctor cleaned the ears with high-pressure water stream; put inside of the ear a tissue with cortisone, done. The ear inflammation was cured within 3 days.
Today the ENT doctors clean the ears with a vacuum pump, giving Antibiotics as drops for the ears and Antibiotic pills. Most of the ear wax remains inside of the ears, and that causes, again and again, an ear inflammation. I could even not swim anymore because I got chronicle ear inflammation.

What to do?

I bought over eBay a syringe for ear cleaning and cleaned the ears by myself,- problem solved.
Then I tried out also 3% Hydrogen Peroxide (3% H2O2) for ear cleaning. And this is even working better. When we have an ear inflammation, we clean with the 3% Hydrogen Peroxide the ears, that is enough, no more medicaments. Hydrogen Peroxide has no side effects, and it will disinfect our ears.

Put it for 5 minutes inside in your ears. Then your hear this sizzle of the hydrogen peroxide. Don't care, without pain no gain. We drain the 3% H2O2 out of the ear. We make this procedure again until there is less sizzle. Done.

What to do if you have Fungus in the ears?

ENT doctors can not heal fungus!

Clean the ears.

Get coconut oil or olive oil, and some garlic cloves. Peel the garlic cloves, cut them one time, cover them with the oil for 24 hours. Put the cloves out, and you have garlic oil. Drop this garlic oil 5 times a day for 5 days inside of your ears, and you will never get fungus again inside of your ears.

My YouTube: How to heal our Ears? https://youtu.be/UwhXzNIjytw

My Audio: https://s3-ap-southeast-1.amazonaws.com/rudizimmerer/2/How+to+heal+our+Ears.mp3

5 Remedies that improve your eyesight

3 Years ago, I had problems with my eyesight and dry eyes… My vision blurred, and often, I could not see sharp…

And today my eyes are better than before, and also my dry eyes are healed…

I have tried out many methods and herbs, including Acupressure and eyesight training.

Most of them didn't work!

Before you try out my remedies, you should consult an eye-doctor because it is forbidden to give any health tip as a non-professional.

1.) Alpha Omega 3 oil for blurred eyesight.
First, I tried out this Fish-oil-supplement as an Alpha Omega 3 Oil, and it didn't work. Afterward, I tried the Flaxseed as an Alpha Omega 3 Oil, and that showed excellent results.

The recent studies found out that the supplement as fish-oil doesn't produce any tangible results … Throw them in the garbage…

The Flaxseed contains an equivalent of the Alpha Omega 3 Oil, and even 30% of the Flaxseed is that precious oil. Get 3 spoon-fool Flaxseed, grind it in a blender, add water to it and wait for 3 -5 minutes. Then consume it with your food.
After one month, your blurred eyesight will improve. Daily consume 3 spoon-full Flaxseed. With the Flaxseed also your digestion will improve.

2.) Wolf-berries from China for better eyesight.

1/2 cub of Wolf-berries soak them in warm water, blend them with an Electric blender, wait 10 minutes, and consume them… Even the 256 Old Chinese herbalist Li Ching-Yuen was eating them every day…

3.) Now comes the scary path - Castor-oil
Castor-oil drastically improves our eye-sight. Results can be seen after one week of using it. It also heals cataract … As usual, what works,- the doctors are against it. Because they lose customers.

The Castor-oil should be pure virgin-oil without any ads …
Get a bottle with an eye-dropper, clean them, cook them out, fill it with the Castor-oil … For 90 days drop 2 drops in each of your eyes, before you go to bed in the night. The oil that spills out rub it with one finger around your eye-lids. If you miss one night, add this one day at the end of the 90 days. After 1 month again you cook out the bottle with the eye-dropper, to kill all bacteria. Keep always the Castor oil in the refrigerator.

4.) Ginkgo Biloba,
is used to heal our eyes and is a remedy for Macular Degeneration. In the future, more than 10% of the population will be blind through Macular Degeneration. The reason is the blue light emitted from the cell-phones, TV and the new electrical light from LED and energy-saving light.

5.) Avoid all blue light. The 6000K light harms us. Try out the 2700K LED-light/ energy-saving light and add some red light as the lighting in your home. On the Cell-phones, PC-displays, and TV should run an App like the F.Lux app or blue light filter app, that reduces the Blue-light.

How to get natural, a more beautiful face?

As I described before, you detox/cleanse your blood, liver and kidneys.
For psoriasis/eczema/acne or other skin problems take the herbs: Yellow dock, burdock, dandelion and nettles. You can make a herbal tea and drink or eat the extract of these herbs.

Normally you take 2 times a day a mixture of all of these herbs or just only one or two of these herbs…

But you should not take more than 2 times of 500mg of the extracted herbs, all together, per day.

I recommend to ask a medical doctor for assistance.

How to heal your face skin and brighten your face skin?

Take 2 cups of water.

Boil the water, then add…

2 Teaspoon green tea.

1 Teaspoon thyme.

1 Teaspoon cinnamon.

Let soak the herbs for 10 minutes.

Filter the ingredients out of the water.

Cool the herbal water down and fill it in an ice cube container.

Put the ice cube container in a freezer, freeze the water.

Take 2 ice cubes.

Put an isolation cotton ball around the ice cubes.

Take the 2 ice cubes one in each hand and hold them with your thumb and index finger…

Rub/ massage with the 2 ice cubes your entire face for 5 minutes.

Then let for 10 minutes dry the herb-water on your face.

Wash your face and put coconut oil or similar on your face.

After 2 hours you can see the awesome results…

Do this for continuously 14 days and your face looks so much better…

How to get rid of wrinkles and skin lines of the face?

If we age our collagen under the skin getting thinner and thinner and our skin is getting loose...

We can actually rebuild the collagen by tapping or with special massage devices…

Some years ago, I bought on eBay a face massage device from China.

It is called Bio-wave photo-ultrasonic galvanic skin care.

Link of a similar device at the end.

Actually, we massage every other day your skin with this device for 7 to 15 minutes, and the skin lines and even some wrinkles get removed.

When we stimulate our skin with tapping, micro current and ultrasound we can rebuild our collagen.

You can try also the normal much stronger electric massage devices for massaging your face and neck… They will work too… But for the sensitive areas around your eyes, you need these special massage devices that I have described before.

Energy Saving Light and LED Bulbs harm our body!

The Energy Saving Light and LED bulbs, LED display emit too much blue light and that harms our body, life expectancy, and can even make us blind. …

The cellular energy or Adenosine triphosphate (ATP) nourish our body cells. Without ATP, we can't live longer than 15seconds.
Our food gives the cells only 30% of the ATP.
With the right light (600 - 1300nm), - the red to infrared light, we can boost our energy. The sun, fire or the old Incandescent bulbs with clear glass, naturally have the red and infrared light. At the end are links with much more information.

The blue light from the Energy Saving Light and LED bulbs, LED/LCD display even disturb our cells so that less ATP is coming to our Cells. This means we harm our body with such unnatural light!!!

In Germany, blindness is caused by 50% from age-related macular degeneration (AMD). The LED screens, LED lamps, and Energy Saving Light Bulbs can cause the AMD.

The natural light from the sun has a whole spectrum light from 0 to 5500K. Fire and the old incandescent bulbs (with clear glass) have a full spectrum light between 0 and 2700K. And the cool white light from the LED and Energy Saving Bulbs have 6500K.

Now here comes a problem we measure colors in Kelvin and in wavelength nm.

The temperature scale is totally different than the wavelength Scale… see the pictures!

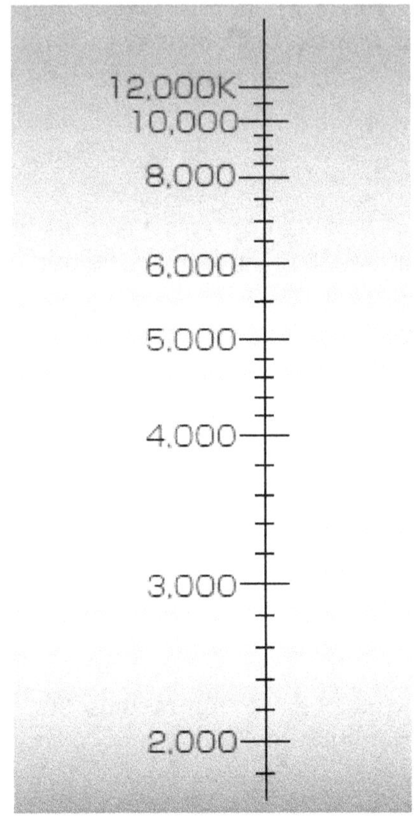

12,000K
10,000
8,000
6,000
5,000
4,000
3,000
2,000

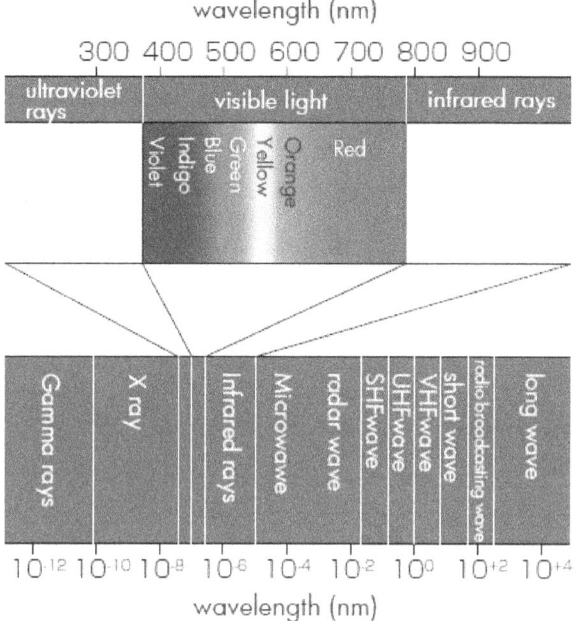

What is infrared light or rays?

Infrared is not heat, nor does it (directly) cause heat; it's emitted by the heat of an object at a specific range of temperatures like the incandescent bulb, fire or even our body. Infrared LED's emit Infrared light without heat. Infrared is not visible for human beings.

The red light is between 600 and 770nm afterward comes the not visible infrared light between 770 and 2000nm.

For our cells is the best light between 600nm and 1300nm.

And this light nourishes our cells.

The magic best light should be the infrared 850nm.

This Infrared light can heal our body and increase our life expectancy. The Infrared light goes through our cloth and can go up to 1 inch inside of our body.

We can buy cheap Infrared LEDs 850nm and a 5Volt power supply from the Internet/eBay/China. Altogether between $10 to 20$. Is this possible?

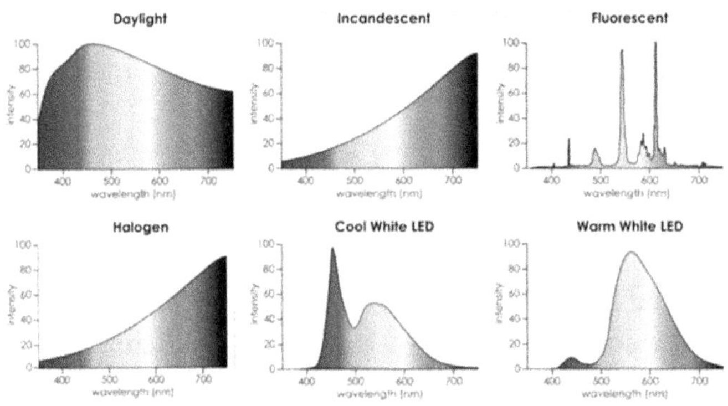

If we compare the whole spectrum from the different light sources, we see that the best light is from the Halogen and Incandescent bulbs with clear glass.

We have the options to buy these old Incandescent bulbs or the 6 to 12V Halogen light with a DC power supply that is the best…. Because a DC power supply doesn't flick the light off and on like the AC current.

I have chosen warm light LED's (2700K), combine it with additionally Red light LEDs and Infrared LEDs. And with this light, I feel really better. For the display of my Laptop, I run the F.Lux app, or we can run the Iris app. With both Apps, we get our red light to the screen.

221

Who wants to read more:
https://articles.mercola.com/sites/articles/archive/2016/10/23/near-infrared-led-lighting.aspx
https://www.facts-are-facts.com/article/energy-saving-light-bulbs-can-make-you-ill

All you want to know about death.

I found an awesome video on YouTube about this topic…

I want to help you to understand and accept death.

A survey of the **Near-Death-Experience** or **NDE** caused by cardiac arrest was made by Dr. Peter Fernwick (his book: the art of dying).

He made a survey of 2000 responses of NDE, from people who never have heard about a NDE before, but had a NDE.

The results are:

A.) The NDE is different from our upbringing, religions, faith, culture. The Western People have more tunnel experience with lights and the Japanese watch to cross a river… Both experiences I never had.

B.) The NDE has a very big impact on our life… My life changed totally and I am grateful for that… Because money, success became meaningless…. Love, happiness, contentment makes more sense!

C.) Is there a consciousness beyond the brain that functions after death?
Yes, this was also for me true. I left just my body and my body is just like a cage or prison…

D.) Is the consciousness beyond the brain? Does our brain filter out information of that consciousness? Or is our consciousness only in the brain?
Science can prove both. But sense makes only that our consciousness is beyond the brain.

E.) Is there a state beyond our duality when we experience death…?
Living in the here and now…?

Absolutely yes, after so many surveys have been done from NDE and dying people in the hospice… I was 3 times already clinically dead. My experience is that I became the neutral witness without judging… Even I saw my dead body and these stupid doctors who had caused my death…. There was no future, past only this moment…

Afterward, Dr. Peter Fernwick made his next survey about the death, interviewed the nurses working in hospices and compared this with other well-known surveys…

What is the dying process in a hospice or in a place where the people can die in peace…

1. 14 days before the death, the deathbed visitors come. These people like to go in your room or stay outside of your room, but they don't like to sit close to you… Because they are scared. For instance, my previous girlfriend has cancer in the third state, she will not die… When I heard that from her, I was scared to be physically close to her… Yes, I thought how lousy I am… then I embraced her…

2. You will realize that you will die and that is shocking.

3. You have to give up your attachments to your spouse, family, wealth… Otherwise, it will hurt a lot! So, the more you are self-centered or have a guild, the more difficult it will be.

4. You have to give up your ego, personal attachment to your body…

5. If you do so, you merge with the universe to get the non-duality…

6. Before you die, you will sit up in your bed, even if you were before paralyzed, or unable… to say bye bye to the visitors.

7. Many nurses (35% of the nurses) have watched flooded light (spiritual light) that fades with the dying.

8. Birds are coming to the window and dogs, cats are howling.

9. Clocks are stopping during the death…

10. Dreams of the dear ones are happening to the dying people. For instance, when my first guru Bhagwan/Osho died, I had my worst nightmares in my entire life. Even I was not his devotee anymore and didn't know that he was dying.

List of 140 Psychosomatic Diseases and How to Cure Them

Today many diseases are caused by eating the wrong food, living in the wrong environment, and relying on western medicine, and medications for diseases, like diabetes. Nevertheless, we should not forget that mainly the cause of diseases are suppressed negative feelings.

I have subdivided the diseases into three categories: reason, suppressed feelings, and actions. For many diseases, the reason and the suppressed feelings are the same. We release the suppressed feelings; just to feel the emotion that caused the diseases or we apply EFT. We need to also accept the disease with its symptoms, which had helped us to integrate a piece of unawareness into our life so that we are becoming more integrated. We should be thankful for this. In the long term, it will enrich our life. When I started this process of self-healing, I was overwhelmed by so many diseases, and I was abusing the symptoms, actually, they worked against me. When I understood that the diseases were to help me, healing occurred. For severe diseases, we need to consult a body and feelings orientated therapist; alone it is too difficult to free us from the traumas. In many cases, an acupressure routine (three labs for one chart and then 5times/day) for a disease will cure it. The first and best acupressure book is from Dr. J. V. Cerney: *Acupressure Without Needles*. Then there is a good Chinese healing book for the eyes, *Healing Your Eyes with Chinese Medicine. Acupuncture, Acupressure & Chinese Herbs*.

There are also many helpful and good mp3 for different diseases from Dr. Steve. G. Jones. Dr. Jones really has the best hypnoses mp3 on the market, and also the biggest selection. How we need to change our food is in the food chapter. I have studied Chi Gong for 30 years, I was able to restore my health mainly from Chi Gong and Acupressure. For this book, I have selected the best Chi Gong exercises. In the chapter about Chi Gong, there are two exercises for the heart, and one exercise to benefit the liver, kidney, pancreas/stomach, and lungs. The list of the psychosomatic diseases is mainly from the German book: *Krankheit als Schlüssel* by best selling author, Dr. Rüdiger Dahlke, M.D. I have added my experience about the healing of different diseases, because, like diabetes, many diseases are dependent on the food that we eat, or can easily be healed with acupressure.

The Meaning and Reason for the Diseases, and

The Action We Need to Take to Heal Ourselves

Abbreviation:
ADA (American Doctor Association) is the highest faculty for American Doctors.

<u>Abscess</u>
Reason: Suppressed deep conflicts want to surface.
Suppressed Feelings: Anger, despair, and grief are coming up, and want to explode.
Action: Express your aggression with full awareness. Go to encounter groups, do the dynamic meditation from Osho, learn boxing.

<u>Acne</u>
Reason: Development of the teenager's sexuality. Fear of sexual surrender to the other gender. The shame of one's own sexuality. The pimples help in trying to be unattractive to the opposite gender.
Suppressed Feelings: Development of the teenager's sexuality. Fear of sexual surrender to the other gender. The shame of one's

own sexuality. The pimples help in trying to be unattractive to the opposite gender.

Action: To embrace and love the other gender. Discover kissing and body sensuality with the other gender. To enjoy your sexuality, share your sexuality with your partner.

Strong Aggressiveness, to go wild about every small thing
Reason: Pent-up anger from the past.
Suppressed Feelings: Pent-up anger from the past.
Action: To learn to communicate and express what you want. Go to encounter groups, do the dynamic meditation from Osho, learn boxing.

Aids
HIV/ AIDS the terrible lie or Business?
Since 1994 I have never believed that Aids exist, because of Leading biochemical scientists, including University of California at Berkeley retrovirus expert Peter Duesberg and Nobel Prize winner Walter Gilbert, have been warning for years that there is no proof that HIV causes AIDS.
http://www.duesberg.com/articles/kmreason.html
Even better Dr. John Bergman proves on science proofed studies that HIV causes AIDS never was true, and just huge business…. Many people got discriminated and killed through very toxic medicaments that never could heal an immune system weakness…or the HIV test could never be verified…. (this you read on every HIV test).

HIV and AIDS- The Real Cause and Solution
Dr. Bergman explains how HIV testing and therapies have never proven accurate or effective and what the real causes and solutions of AIDS are. Actually aids doesn't exist or is not caused through hiv… see the video:
https://www.youtube.com/watch?v=hD8p-M8qgP0

Reason:

Suppressed love and sex without feelings, too much sex for the body, so that the immune system got weak.

Suppressed Feelings: Fear to love, to open the heart, to get rejected and to get hurt.

Action: Open the heart and start to love somebody with all your passion, regardless if you might get hurt, or rejected. Dr. Robert O. Becker discovered that with electrical current you can kill all viruses in the blood.

http://www.abovetopsecret.com/forum/thread585556/pg1

http://www.silentcures.com/AIDS-CURES-THAT-WORK.html

Allergy

Reason: To defense inside again something with all of your aggression

Suppressed Feelings: Strong Aggression against your surrounding environment. Fear for life, vitality, sex, lust, love; for things you can't control that are overwhelming for you.

Action: Learn to say no, when you are asked to do volunteer or say no to spending time with people you don't like. Learn to express anger. Accept your anger as a part of yourself. Do and experience the things that you are afraid of. Go to encounter groups, do the dynamic meditation from Osho, learn boxing.

Alzheimer/Dementia disease

Reason: To escape from the present and don't want to take any more responsibility; because life is too difficult. The main reason for Alzheimers is that people are taking too many medications. (According to the ADA: if you take more than 3 medications, then the risk of developing dementia is twice as high). If we know that an older relative takes a lot of medications, then we can predict that dementia is around the corner.

Suppressed Feelings: Fear of aging and conflicts of every kind.

Action: Try to live in the here and now. Relax, try taking small steps to get involved and engaged again with the world and your surroundings. Stop all kinds of medications if possible. Do a complete detox, and become a vegan.

Amnesia
Reason: To escape from the past.
Suppressed Feelings: Fear to bear the responsibility of your actions, or because you can't bear memories of the past.
Action: Learn to trust, and to let go.

Amenorrhea, lack of menstruation.
Reason: Anorexia, stress, sadness, malnourishment, and over stimulation
Suppressed Feelings: You weren't able to be a carefree child when you were younger, you have not experienced all those feelings.
Action: Go back to your childhood and really be a child. The way to do this is to be a babysitter and play with children, and follow them and participate in their childish games.

Anemia
Reason: Not enough color or passion in life.
Suppressed Feelings: Vitality, spontaneity, fear to live a life full of passion.
Action: To relax; begin to do meditation; to find calmness inside of yourself. And then start to express yourself out in the world. Start to join groups for expressing yourself; encounter groups and bioenergetic groups are good for this. Continue to work on your feelings of calmness, so that you have both parts of you, a still and silent part, and a vital and vibrant part.

Apathy
Reason: Refusal to live and to participate in life.
Suppressed Feelings: Fear of sorrow.
Action: Learn to meditate and find stillness inside of yourself. Then come back to the world.

Appendicitis

Reason: War, conflict in the subconscious mind , the inability to process hard conflicts.

Suppressed Feelings: Feelings seem to lead to a dead end. Strong aggression wants to surface.

Action: Understand that you at a dead end at this, and just accept your inability to continue living in this manner.

Lack of Appetite
Reason: Refusal to live and to participate in life.

Suppressed Feelings: Refusal to live and to participate in life.

Action: Try to fast for some days, meditate, and start again to live.

Adenoid Childhood Polyps
Reason: To have the nasal passages blocked; can't breathe through the nose. To have too many conflicts.

Suppressed Feelings: It is excessive demand and frustration.

Action: Go inside yourself to look for conflicts, and wait until you are ready and then open again to the world. Be more confident and say what you need and what you don't want.

Arthrosis
Reason: Too much meat, too little raw foods.

Suppressed Feelings:?

Action: Detox the body with fasting; become a vegan and eat raw foods. See the Food Chapter and Prevention Chapter.

Asthma
Reason: Deep Traumas. Fear of losing freedom; fear to give and not get back; fear to become dependent. Be aggressive towards others, and use asthma to make others feel sorry for you so that you get the things you want.

Suppressed Feelings: Deep fear or aggression

Action: Breathing exercise/therapy and sports. Exercise: climbing stairs. Go to a body and feelings orientated therapist and work on your suppressed traumas, most of the time they are issues from your childhood. I don't think you can solve the problem alone without a therapist.

Barleycorn; sty
Reason: There is a conflict that stabs the eye, whether we face the conflict or don't face the conflict.
Suppressed Feelings:?
Action: Learn to face the conflict and also to let go of a conflict that is burning the eye. Put warm chamomile tea bags on your eyes to soothe them.

Bed-wetting
Reason: We want to release our tension and stress, and the pressure we feel, and this is only possible for us during the night.
Suppressed Feelings: Sadness, frustration.
Action: A note for the parents, don't put too much pressure on your child! Let your child relax and cry as often he/she wants. Give your child freedom. For the child: express your feelings much more. For more information, consult the book: *Acupressure Without Needles*. Acupressure is recommended for Bedwetting, it will solve the problem.

Cystitis, inflammation of the bladder
Reason: Too long sitting on a cold surface. Conflicts - an internal war between letting go of the conflict or not.
Suppressed Feelings: Conflicts
Action: Learn to let go of old problems that you can't solve.

Bladder cancer
Reason: Suppressed conflicts over a long time period, mostly from childhood. The wrong things to eat are acidic foods.
Suppressed Feelings:
Action: Go to a body and feelings orientated therapist and work on your suppressed sadness and traumas, most of the time it is coming from your childhood. I don't believe that you can solve the

problem alone without a therapist. Also, change the foods that you eat.

Bladder stones
Reason: Food has too much acid. Not drinking enough distilled water (2 liter/day). Holding onto problems too long, instead of letting them go!
Suppressed Feelings: Holding onto old problems.
Action: Change food, Drink 2 liter/day of distilled water, learn to forgive, and to let go of problems.

Blindness, being able to see less than 10%
Reason: We don't want to face our issues, so we must look inside of ourselves.
Suppressed Feelings: Fear of our inner and outer world.
Action: To accept our blindness and to start our journey working on our inner selves.

Blood Clot, Thrombosis
Reason: You are eating the wrong foods. You need to detox because the body is too acidic. Start with fresh fruit and vegetable juice. Become a vegan and eat raw food. Fruits clean the blood vessels when eaten on an empty stomach. Also, do exercises and be active after you have consumed fruits and fruit juice.
Suppressed Feelings: ?
Action: ?

Low blood pressure
Reason: You don't want to live your life fully.
Suppressed Feelings: You have fears about living your life fully.
Action: Read this book: *Acupressure Without Needles*. Try acupressure for low blood pressure, it will solve the problem.

Bowel diseases
Reason: The biggest issue is eating the wrong foods, and taking medications that destroy the balance between beneficial and non

beneficial bacteria in the bowels (85% to 15%). Another contributing factor is not enough fiber in the foods you eat. You are not getting enough exercise for your body, and you have too much fear.

Suppressed Feelings: All kinds of feelings, and especially fear.

Action: Change your lifestyle, eat the right food, and add raw fermented vegetables to your diet. You can read more about fermented foods and eating the right foods in the food chapter, also daily exercise for your body and massage your bowels.

Brain tumor

Reason: Your thinking is beyond your nature and your feelings. It causes you to suppress your nature, temperament, and feelings. In other words, you think that you are your thinking and that you are not your nature or subconsciousness. The best example is Brendon Burchard! He is beyond his subconsciousness (after a discussion with him!). He thinks that he is capable of higher thinking, so eventually, he got a brain tumor.

Suppressed Feelings: All kinds of Feelings.

Action: Go to a body and feelings orientated therapist and work on this issue of a tumor. I don't think you can solve the problem alone without a therapist. And then feel and live your nature. Don't overload your head with thinking, begin to feel your negative feelings, and don't think that you don't have negative feelings like Brendon Burchard!

Breast cancer

The breast is a symbol of motherhood, feeding, security, sensuality, and sexuality.

Reason: Fear to live your femininity, to be a woman and mother. You are shy about being a woman. You try to refuse that you are a woman.

Suppressed Feelings: femininity, motherhood, sexuality

Action: Be and live your life as a woman, regardless if others love or accept it. You were born as a strong woman, so be that woman. Find your mothering instinct inside of you, live your sexuality. Pay attention to how other feminine women live and express their feelings. Then try it out in your own way to embrace your femininity and be a woman. Every day, massage your breasts; Learn about Mantak Chia and Tao love. Go to a body and feelings orientated therapist and work on your suppressed traumas, most of the time they come from your childhood. I don't think that you can solve the problem alone without a therapist.

Breast cyst
Reason: Irritated hormone system, you are not in balance
Suppressed Feelings: Hurt feelings during pregnancy, or during breastfeeding. You feel that you are not a good enough mother. You don't pay enough attention to your feelings, you don't offer yourself enough love or care.
Action: To take care good of yourself, and love yourself. Love yourself. Massage your breast every day; try Mantak Chia and Tao love. Go to a body and feelings orientated therapist and work on your suppressed traumas, most of the time they come from your childhood. I don't think that you can solve the problem alone without a therapist.

Bronchitis
Reason: You are not aware of the being that is inside of you so that you can't express it outside of you.
Suppressed Feelings: Doubts, and critical thoughts.
Action: To learn to express your thoughts and feelings, read this book: *Acupressure Without Needles*. Do acupressure treatment for bronchitis and your problem is solved.

Burn-out-Syndrome
Reason: The feeling that you are no longer productive or getting enough done or that you are not good enough. You are a self exploiter.
Suppressed Feelings: Escape from an overwhelming situation.
Action: Take a vacation and then understand that nothing is under our control. We need to do what we can do, that is good enough

and we don't need to be perfect. The more tension and stress we are under, the less effective we are. Good is enough. Make a perfect plan to have enough time for pleasure, rest, and love.

Bulimia

Reason: Refusal to become a woman. The inability to accept your own feminine body. You are trying to escape the inner emptiness by filling up the stomach. You then punish this eating with puking and with fasting. You like to be pure, and strong; you want to be an ascetic and to have all your feelings and thoughts under control.

Suppressed Feelings: Fear of orgasms, of masturbation, and of enjoying your own sensuality and sexuality. In the time period of fasting, you want to conquer the spiritual world, and in a period of excess eating, you like to conquer the mundane world.

Action: Discover your new feminine body. Enjoy being a woman, enjoy your body through masturbation, orgasms, sensuality, and sexuality as often as you like. Be sexual and express your feelings that way instead of eating like crazy and then fasting like crazy. Read sex journals and erotica for inspiration.

Buxism

Reason: Tension; suppressed anger; huge resistance against the current situation.

Suppressed Feelings: Aggression

Action: Release the tension and aggression; learn to defend yourself; learn to say no; learn to show your aggression; train your endurance, don't give up.

Cardiovascular problems

Reason: Blood pressure is too low, sensitivity to changes in the weather; for big guys, this is quite normal.

Suppressed Feelings:

Action: Exercise like jogging, cycling, and swimming are good for your body. Instead of drinking coffee, exercise until you feel good, and full of energy. For low blood pressure try acupressure. Don't use the elevator, climb the stairs.

Cataract

Reason: Unclear, blurred vision. We don't like to see sharp reality, the harsh truth is too much, we can see only a bad future without hope and faith.

Suppressed Feelings: Fear of getting older or new perspectives.

Action: Get rid of your negativity so that you have a more positive perspective on life. Release the negativity. See this book for inspiration: *Healing Your Eyes with Chinese Medicine. Acupuncture, Acupressure &Chinese Herbs.*

Chronic Fatigue Syndrome

Reason: To be too weak and tired, so that after your workday, you are too exhausted to do anything fun, or to take care of household chores. Aggressive self-destructive thoughts and behaviors; to weaken the nerve system.

Suppressed Feelings: Depression

Action: Read this book: *Acupressure Without Needles.* Try acupressure for healing. Try to find what you want in your life. And believe that you can achieve it. Read motivational books.

Claustrophobia

Reason: The trauma of birth has not been processed consciously.

Suppressed Feelings: Fear

Action: Go to a body and feelings orientated therapist, and work on your birth trauma. I don't think you can solve the problem alone without a therapist.

Colon inflammation and other problems

Reason: There is a big war in the subconsciousness.

Suppressed Feelings:

Action: Try a feelings and body orientated therapy, like Bio dynamic, or Bio Energetic. For the food: choose to become a vegan. Change your diet: eat vegetables and potatoes; on a empty stomach eat raw fruits, then after a half hour you can eat again; have blended fruits with green leaves as a green smoothie, and fruit

and vegetable juice; now comes the super trick: eat unpasteurized fermented vegetables, which will replace the bad bacteria with good bacteria so that your colon will heal.   See Dr. John Bergman
https://www.youtube.com/watch?v=TiigsFnNDuQ
Do a colon cleanse from Blessed Herbs
http://www.blessedherbs.com/products/cleansing-detox-kits.html
This is a so great detox and helps for our colon
And afterward, eat fermented vegetables every day. See the chapter about food.
Try an inner organ massage from Mantak Chia
http://www.universal-tao.com/ It is so good to keep our colon young and healthy. I do this massage every day for 5 minutes.

Common cold
Reason: To need a break from the world, too many conflicts, and want a barrier from the outside world. Change to cool weather/season and to be inflexible to adapt to it.
Suppressed Feelings: Aggression
Action: Escape and be alone for a time to recharge, until you can be open again to the world. Read this book: *Acupressure Without Needles*. Try acupressure for the common cold, and the problem is solved. Prepare yourself for the cool weather/season change. You feel/imagine the cold weather before it happens.

Conjunctivitis
Reason: We don't like to confront/see conflict, like the ostrich, we want to dig our head in the sand when we are feeling overwhelmed.
Suppressed Feelings: Fear, overwhelmed by conflict.
Action: Take a rest, relax and then confront the issue again.

Corn, wart, callus on the foot
Reason: There is an energy reflex point for every organ on our foot. Look up the area and find the reflex point of the organ. If this corn/wart/callus is hurting. then there is something wrong with this organ. Or your shoes are too small for your feet.

Suppressed Feelings:
Action: Wear more comfortable shoes. Massage this point and make sure that you heal this organ corresponding to the reflex point.

Deafness
Reason: To exclude yourself from the world; like to be alone; like to disobey; to close up your heart.
Suppressed Feelings: Overwhelmed
Action: To go inside and find the stillness inside of yourself. To find inner peace and then you can start to communicate again.

Sudden deafness, acute hearing loss
Reason: Through excessive demand/stress to close the ears, shut yourself away from the world.
Suppressed Feelings: Fear of stress, to be overwhelmed.
Action: Take yourself away from the world, release your stress and then come back.

Dementia see Alzheimer disease

Depression
Reason: suppressed anger and life energy that is directed against ourselves, an extreme is a tendency towards suicide.
Suppressed Feelings: Sadness, anger, fear to take responsibility.
Action: Therapy, or releasing the suppressed feelings with EFT. Sport and exercise to gain back the energy, to have the power to feel, to release the suppressed feelings. My experience as a therapist is that exercise to build strength immediately brings the suppressed feelings up. Then you can let them go. Easy!

Dermatitis
Reason: Problems to get in touch with the world/people.
Suppressed Feelings: Fear of getting hurt, or being rejected by people.

Action: To overcome the own barrier, to seek out contact with the world/people.

Diabetes See the Chapter about diabetes and see the pancreas.

Diarrhea
Reason: Fear or tropical bacteria.
Suppressed Feelings: Fear
Action: Release the fear. Take no medications! Fasting for some days until it is gone or eating bananas or rusk, and drinking black tea without sugar/milk. Build up the right bacteria when the diarrhea is gone with unpasteurized fermented vegetables (5Tbs/day is enough) for 4 weeks.
Diarrhea is a good detox for the body.

Dyslexia
Reason: The dyslexics use the right side (instead of the left side of the brain) for reading and writing, many also for speaking, me too. I also have dyslexia. So that we can't see the logic in writing, we only have our feelings and memory for reading and writing. And we need an editor! The good thing is that many creative people are dyslexic like Richard Branson.
Suppressed Feelings:
Action: Support dyslexia in creativity instead of nagging about their poor writing.

Dyspareunia
Reason: Refusal of sex with a male.
Suppressed Feelings: Fear of sex, or surrender to a loved one. Trauma of a past rape; bad lover; reason for not wanting to have sex.
Action: Learn to say no, learn to surrender to love, learn to enjoy sex with a male. Let go of the trauma. Begin feelings and body orientated therapy, like Biodynamic, or Bioenergetic.

Epilepsy

Reason: A huge inner (electrical) tension is released in our brain so that all the fuses are blown/shut off. This is an epilepsy attack. This released energy causes cramps in our body (I also had epilepsy) and we lose consciousness. We have tried to control our feelings and thoughts too much so that these attacks are happening. I got the epilepsy attacks through the self-conditioning of my mind and suppressing my anger.

Suppressed Feelings: Anger

Action: Participate in an Encounter and Bioenergetic group, Practice the Dynamic Meditation from Osho on a daily basis. Work at it so that you really feel and release your anger, and then there is no reason for epilepsy anymore. I have done this and been successful, I have not had an attack or any headaches for 35 years!

Esophageal cancer

Reason: Smoking and unhealthy lifestyle.

Suppressed Feelings: ?

Action: Fasting and then changing to a healthy raw food diet. See the chapter about cancer, prevention, and food.

Facial nerve paresis

Reason: One-sidedness, the two different faces of a human being. Goethe calls this concept two souls in the breast. In most of the cases, it is the left side of the face that is paralyzed. This means the suppression of the female feelings of your being, including sadness, tenderness, and love .

Suppressed Feelings: The left side of the face is paralyzed: which corresponds to female feelings; the right side of the face corresponds to male feelings.

Action: As fast as possible, get acupuncture treatments, and make faces 3/day in front of the mirror. I had this issue in the past too.

Farsightedness

Reason: Don't want to see the details, or the small stuff, and want to keep the overall view while sacrificing the details. Aging.

Suppressed Feelings:

Action: As you are aging, make sure to exercise your eyes every day so that you don't lose short-sightedness. I make sure to do this every day. Have an objective overview of your life. Make your goal list. Get unattached from life circumstances.

Food intolerance

Reason: Protest or war against the world; the food intolerance shows that you consider the world as your enemy.

Suppressed Feelings: Aggression against everything in front of you.

Action: Confrontation with everything that is strange. Exhaust yourself going through the polarities with the things that you like or don't like until you see the world as one.

Frigidity

Reason: Fear of sexuality, fear of orgasms and losing control during orgasms, past history of rape, fear of men, aggression against sex.

Suppressed Feelings:

Action: Body and feelings orientated therapy, Tantric groups. I don't believe that you can solve the problem alone without a therapist. There are some traumas that you experienced before. The trauma might even be from when you were an infant.

Food addiction, binge eating

Reason: Not getting enough of what you need; you feel empty.

Suppressed Feelings: Hungry for love, love of life.

Action: To live that love, that pleasure, that you really want and not to substitute it with food.

Gall bladder inflammation, cancer, stones, colic

Reason: Suppressed anger.

Suppressed Feelings:

Action: Let your anger out, choose a healthy way such as boxing, martial arts, sports, encounter, or bioenergetic. For gall bladder stones, do a liver cleansing, see more information at the end of the book.

Glaucoma

Reason: Painful eyes, high pressure in your eyes. It comes from too many disappointments, too much sadness, emotional pain from the past, all of this produces the pressure in the eyes.

Suppressed Feelings: Emotional pain, including unreleased sadness, that is insufficient crying and tears to release pain.

Action: Go to a body and feelings orientated therapist and work on your suppressed sadness and traumas. I don't think you can solve the problem alone without a therapist. Because there are traumas that caused it.

Gout

Reason: Eating the wrong food, the body is too acidic from eating meat.

Suppressed Feelings:

Action: Fasting, see the chapter about food..

Gum bleeding

Reason: Damaged or low self-confidence.

Suppressed Feelings:

Action: Explore inside yourself to really see what the reason is for your lack of confidence and then recognize your strength and good habits. Build up your self-esteem. Use an oral irrigator for cleaning your teeth.

Hardness of hearing

Reason: Try to separate/distance yourself from the world; perhaps you don't want to obey the rules that others obey; you don't want to hear anymore, maybe your surroundings are too loud or too exhausting; you show signs of inflexibility, and you are conservative.

Suppressed Feelings: Overwhelmed

Action: Distance yourself from the world to open up to the inner spiritual world. Look inside yourself, instead of refusing the outside environment.

Heart attack or other heart diseases.
Reason: Too much stress, eating the wrong food, wrong medications, and not enough physical exercise. As you can read in my chapter about the heart, a raw foods eater can't get a heart attack but they could have a heart rhythms attack.
Suppressed Feelings:
Action: See my chapter about heart problems.

Hemorrhoids
Reason: Too much sitting and not enough exercise. You have a problem letting go of the problems that you can't solve. You have a fear of expressing your own opinions.
Suppressed Feelings:
Action: Learn to let go of problems and have the courage to say unpopular things. Shave your bottom every week and clean it with water after using the toilet.

Hand sweat or wet hands
Reason: Fear of rejection, and fear of contact with others. Many times there is a fear of sex.
Suppressed Feelings: Fear
Action: Face your fears.

Headache
Reason: To live too much in your head; trying to solve feelings through thinking; to block thoughts-impulses; high-pressure situations where we attempt to think about solutions instead of relaxing; you are too intellectual instead of living through the heart; to be too inflexible in your thinking; not being able to let go of problems; trying to keep everything under your control; desperately looking for a solution; perfectionism. Fear is driving the thoughts 80% of the time.

Suppressed Feelings: Fear
Action: Have more trust in your gut feelings; learn to relax and to let go, don't try to be perfect just be good enough for now, later you can improve on it; trust and have faith instead of thinking constantly; learn to live in your heart. For more information, see Dr. Steve G. Jones' hypnotherapy mp3.

Hypersomnia

Reason: Excess demand; fear of demand from outside. Escape into the dream world.
Suppressed Feelings: Fear
Action: Go to a body and feelings orientated therapist and work on your childhood. I don't think you can solve the problem alone without a therapist.

Hypoglycemia

Reason: Not enough sugar in the blood, it means you have too little sweetness and love in your life.
Suppressed Feelings: Fear/ sadness not getting enough love/happiness
Action: To decide that your life is not fulfilling and that you deserve more.

Impotence

Reason: Fear of death, orgasms, and losing control. Fear about being a man, having aggression, the pressure to perform, fear of not getting an erection, fear of rejection from the female, fear of being a failure and of sexuality. To view sexuality as dirty and to have a bad consciousness.
Suppressed Feelings:
Action: Release all the fears with EFT. Focus your life on love and not so much on sexuality. When you really love someone then the lust will come. If you focus only on sex, then for sure you will fail, instead, focus on loving the woman.

Incontinence

Reason: Fear. The desire to have control over your life is now in the opposite direction. You become again a baby with diapers.
Suppressed Feelings: Deep fear.
Action: Go to a body and feelings orientated therapist and work on your suppressed fears and traumas, most of the time they are coming from your childhood. I don't think you can solve the problem alone without a therapist.

Indigestion
Reason: Disturbance that we can't digest: impressions (travel, new environment) from outside; assimilation of the impression; excretion of the impressions.
Suppressed Feelings:
Action: We prepare for a new scene, or environment; we give ourselves time to digest the new impressions; then we can let go of them faster.

Inflammation
Reason: A conflict, or war, aggression against something.
Suppressed Feelings: If you don't get irritated, annoyed, or angry in your consciousness about something you care about, then you get inflammation somewhere in your body.
Action: If we take antibiotics for that, then we can't solve the root of the problem. So look inside and release the suppressed feelings. Over 2 years, every 6 weeks I had angina, sinusitis, or frontal sinusitis when I took antibiotics. It was a nightmare and then I decided never to take antibiotics again for such diseases. And it was cured by itself, and I never got it again! Still, every year, I get an ear inflammation from swimming. Again I stopped taking antibiotics, still I have to get my ears cleaned by the doctor or I do it myself. And then I wait a week until it is cured by itself. The only antidote that can be used as a substitute for an antibiotic, that doesn't kill the bacteria in our bowel is **colloidal silver**. If this works for you fine. If I get a tooth root inflammation then I take colloidal silver for 10 days, at the dosage of 2 Tbs/day.

Inflammation of the cornea, keratitis
Reason: Not willing to see the reality of wanting to ignore reality, in order not to get angry or sad. You ignore the things that are happening against your will.
Suppressed Feelings: Fear of the reality/conflicts that are against you.
Action: To decide that you want to see what is there and not to be involved anymore in seeing only the things that you desire. Also, begin working on your suppressed fears.

Insomnia
Reason: Through diseases, including the bladder, heart, and pain. Unsolved problems, perfect-isms.
Suppressed Feelings: Fear from unsolved problems.
Action: Sleeping Hypnosis is a helpful mp3 (Dr. Steve G. Jones). Solve your problems in small doable steps. Make a to do list every night about what you want to do the next day. After the 80/20% rule (20% of the activities bring 80% of the results, the other 80% of the activities we can let go) prioritize the tasks. Let go of the problems that you can't solve. Make an anxiety list with all the fear aspects of the problem that you can't solve, prioritize them and then the fears are gone. Let go of perfectionism, believe that good is good enough.

Kidney inflammation and diseases
Reason: War of the inner differences/polarities/opposites (for instance: female and male), partnerships, problems. Wrong Food, too much acidic food, coffee (to process 1 cup of coffee, the kidney needs 24 hours), too many spices and salt is poison for the kidneys. I have met many motorcyclists who get kidney inflammation just from a motorbike ride without a kidney belt and this happens even in the summertime!
Suppressed Feelings: After Chinese Healing: a deep fear
Action: To face the problems in their polarity, so that we really understand what is happening inside of us. For instance, we have an inner child inside of us (the 3-year-old child that wants pleasure,

fun, playtime, and is protesting against every pressure) and the superego (our 6-year-old child that wants to fit into the society). This means we need playtime (3 yrs child) and time to work (6 yrs child)! If one side doesn't get enough, then there is an imbalance and there will be protesting. Change your food. Drink a lot of distilled water, up to 4 to 5 liters per day if possible. Afterward, keep drinking water (2 liters/day). Keep your kidneys warm.

Kidney stones
Reason: Fossilized feelings, themes, and problems are hoarded inside of you instead of letting them go. Or too many acidic foods and not drinking enough water are producing the stones.
Suppressed Feelings:
Action: Begin to experience these old undigested feelings again, work through the themes and then let them go. Learn to forgive and start to live and love again.

Lack of sexual drive
Reason: Too much stress, work, problems, lack of money, tension through your career, tension with the spouse. Bad consciousness about sex, sex is too boring. Fear of getting pregnant, or getting sexual diseases. Taking the wrong medications like beta-blockers. A history of sexual abuse. A hormone imbalance.
Suppressed Feelings:
Action: To value sex, and the erotic. Look for a better form of pregnancy prevention. Learn Tantric. Do a colon cleaning from Blessed Herbs. Detoxing the bowels increases the libido. Also, raw fermented vegetables is a great detox for the bowels.

Liver inflammation, hepatitis, diseases
Reason: For Chinese healing: The reason is anger. Anger for intolerance, or for conservative destructive judging. Too many drugs. Eating the wrong food that is too acidic, or too greasy.
Suppressed Feelings: Anger.
Action: Try Chi Gong. For your liver health, release all the old suppressed anger and develop compassion for everybody. Stop

taking drugs. Change your food, see the food chapter and Chi Gong chapter for more information.

Lumbago

Reason: Fight against yourself. A change in your environment, like moving to a new place or a new job. Taking on a new challenge.

Suppressed Feelings: Aggression and fear of something that you don't want, and at the same time want. Feelings of ambivalence.

Action: Accept and feel your ambivalence, communicate with the different voices inside of you, with the voices which want the change and the voices that hate the change . Relax, and go for a massage.

Lungs diseases

Reason: Sadness, Depression. Smoking.

Suppressed Feelings:

Action: We have to support the immune system. Then we must release the old suppressed feelings. This can be done through acupressure and doing Chi Gong.

Menstruation pain

Reason: Sexual problems; lack of surrender to sex and love; anger that you cannot get pregnant.

Suppressed Feelings:

Action: To accept womanhood, to love your female body instead of rejecting it.

Menstruation too weak, bleeding without egg,

Reason: Not enough femininity, lack of a desire to have a child.

Suppressed Feelings: Rejection of your femininity.

Action: To feel your motherhood instinct inside of yourself, to be a mature female, to love to have children.

Migraine

Reason: One sidedness in thinking and feelings; fear of failure; insult of feminine self-esteem; paying for your closed up feelings with migraine headaches; conflict between thinking and sexual drive (try to live your sexuality in your head or to suppress your sexuality in your head); to blackmail people with your migraine.
Suppressed Feelings:
Action: To pacify your sexuality with your thinking (live your sexuality and don't live it only in your head); stop using your migraine to blackmail people; balance your feelings with your thinking.

Miscarriage
Reason: You don't want the child or you are under too much stress (the wrong environment, wrong father).
Suppressed Feelings:
Action: Go to a body and feelings orientated therapist and work on this trauma! Otherwise, you will carry this trauma your whole life. And then you won't be able to ever accept children. Accept the fact of your miscarriage, we are not perfect. My partner and I had two miscarriages, so I know how hard that is!

Multiple Sclerosis
Reason: Too much self -discipline; suppressing the sexual drive, freedom, happiness, vitality, sensuality; aggression that is directed against yourself; desire to plan everything in your life even when it is not under your control; to be inflexible and think that only your way of thinking and handling a situation is right (perhaps you have learned this way of thinking from your parents, so it is not yours); to ignore your own demands and to fulfill other demands. A clear 'No' to yourself; strong resistance against loving yourself, accepting yourself, and forgiving yourself. You are very hard on yourself, you never treat yourself with compassion, you refuse expressing softness; deep down you hate yourself!
Suppressed Feelings:
Action: To love yourself with all of your errors, to become soft and flexible, to be in a state of flux. Go to a body and feelings

orientated therapist and work on your traumas, and begin to live. I don't think you can solve the problem alone without a therapist. You can never make it alone. I have seen MS patients, like this, they are so hard and to make them soft takes years of therapy.

Nail chewing

Reason: Fear and guilty feelings about expressing the anger that is inside. This way, the anger remains inside and the weapon, the nails, is getting defused.
Suppressed Feelings: Fear about expressing anger.
Action: To be more active in your life, and to use anger for being productive in your life. Otherwise, express the anger.

Nausea/to puke

Reason: Not enough acceptance; you take something in but don't want to digest it, and you end up throwing it out.
Suppressed Feelings: A conflict/ situation that we don't want to digest.
Action: To accept your own resistance, to protest if it is necessary, if not then feel the resistance inside of yourself.

Neck stiffness

Reason: Stubbornness, pigheadedness, persistence. To go through the world with blinders on, you don't want to see all aspects of a situation, you believe that only your view is right.
Suppressed Feelings:
Action: Focus is great and to see the whole picture is even better! Begin to open up to all sides and remain focused on your goal.

Necrospermia, the immovability of the semen (sterility)

Reason: Toxic food, pollution, and western medicine. To be too much a man of action. Don't want to procreate.
Suppressed Feelings:
Action: Take a vacation, relax, and learn to meditate.

Neurodermatitis

Reason: Fight inside of the person against building up hostile images, strong and unaware of aggression.
Suppressed Feelings: Pent up aggression, vitality
Action: Go to a body and feelings orientated therapist and work on your traumas, such as aggression. I don't think you can solve the problem alone without a therapist, because the aggression is unconscious. Try to open your borders and really feel what is coming inside. Try to live more, have the courage to do the things that you want. Decide to take the challenges instead of getting overwhelmed from by them. Be more aggressive so that you don't need the Neurodermatitis. My girl friend took 14 days of Thai herbs from a Thai herb doctor in Krabi, then the Neurodermatitis was gone/healed.

Orgasm problems

Reason: Men have more orgasm problems then women, because ejaculation doesn't necessarily mean an orgasm. In an orgasm, the whole body is involved, it includes strong breathing; both partners are moving together in unison and moaning. It should be moments of ecstasy. Fear of losing control and letting the body take control. Fear of rejection from your partner, fear of enjoying sex.
Suppressed Feelings: Fear of sexuality, fear of losing control, fear of rejection, bad consciousness, afraid to enjoy sex.
Action: Try therapy, Tantra, or encounter groups. Solve the problem on your own is rarely possible.

Osteoporosis

Reason: Eating food that is too acidic and not enough physical exercise. Inside you lose your power, stability, and security. After age 50, you want to get rid of what is not needed, you begin to prepare for death.
Suppressed Feelings:
Action: Begin to get rid of all the things/securities that are not needed anymore including the body's excess weight. Then build up new structures in your life.

Ovarian insufficiency
Reason: Rejected femininity, fear of being a complete woman.
Suppressed Feelings:
Action: Become a woman and appreciate it; love your sensuality, sexuality, you're your femininity.

Ovaritis, oophoritis
Reason: Inner conflict about having a child.
Suppressed Feelings: Fear of carrying out the responsibility of being a mother, inner struggle between wanting and not wanting a child. Anger at one's self for making the right decision.
Action: Release the tension and suppressed feelings. Consider all the opportunities to be a mother and decide what is best for yourself.

Ovarian insufficiency
Reason: Don't want to have a child, too many problems, wrong partner.
Suppressed Feelings: Fear of having a child, or fear of bonding with a child.
Action: Think over your life. What is important for you? Is career more important than being female? Do you think that as a female, you have a better chance at success in your career when you are suppressing your femininity?

Overactive Thyroid Gland.
Reason: Too much vitality; the insatiable appetite for life; over-eager; over demanding; fear of missing something; over alertness; authority conflict; self-denial; not getting enough recognition from the family; avoiding cramped situations.
Suppressed Feelings: Fear of Death. Escape of life, happiness, and love in order to reach your goals.
Action: Live your ambitions; don't allow others to stop you or let yourself get discouraged; be aware that your fear of death is your driving force. Confront yourself with the death of your

imagination, so that you lose the fear of death. Relax and enjoy your life, instead of always running after something.

Pancreas diseases

Today's processed food is poison for the pancreas. See the chapter about diabetes and food.

After Chinese Healing, the suppressed or negative feelings of the pancreas are worry and to see life too seriously. The virtues are fairness and openness. We feel our worry and then develop the virtues of fairness and openness. In the chapter about Chi Gong, we learn an exercise for the pancreas.

Parkinson disease

Reason: Forced stillness causes the trembling. Paralyzed: The excess will cause the inability to move. Fear of death or overwhelming anger can cause trembling. A discrepancy between what you want and what is possible. Too much acidic food.

Suppressed Feelings: Fear and Anger, the thirst for power.

Action: Take a retreat, and process what you have accomplished already in the world. Appreciate the small things in life, instead of only paying attention to the big things. The small things that we are. (Oscar Wild). To face the possibility of death and be at peace with it. Change your food, see food chapter.

Paruresis and shy bladder

Reason: Tension through fear; fear of masculinity for a teenager; fear of letting go; shame and embarrassment while using public toilets.

Suppressed Feelings:

Action: Be proud to be a man, enjoy your sexuality, enjoy letting go.

Pleurisy, pleuritis

Reason: Conflict to communicate.

Suppressed Feelings:

Action: Say honestly what you think and feel.

Pneumonia

Reason: It is a weakness of our immune system, 50% of the population already have the Pneumokokken in their lungs. Chinese Healing believes that diseases of the lungs are caused through sadness and depression.

Suppressed Feelings: Sadness, Depression.

Action: It is a problem that the antibiotic is not strong enough anymore for every pneumonia. We have to support the immune system. Then release the old suppressed feelings. Try acupressure and Chi Gong.

Pregnancy-related-problems

Reason: Unconsciously not wanting to be pregnant, not wanting to carry the baby to term. When she throws up, she is trying to throw up the fetus.

Suppressed Feelings: Wanting to get rid of the fetus.

Action: Take time to process all the ambivalent feelings you have about becoming a mother. Prepare yourself to become a mother. For instance, when I prepared myself inside for the cold winter, I didn't catch a cold in the wintertime.

Premature ejaculation

Reason: Fear of being a bad lover, too much tension, too much sexual pressure, fear of failure, you don't love your partner, you don't want to have sex.

Suppressed Feelings:

Action: Let go of the tension. Play sports or workout before sex, meditate, get a massage, relax, release the sexual tension with masturbation before having sex. Breathe deeply in and out, feel it in your whole body when you penetrate your partner. Read the book: *Acupressure without needles*. Try acupressure for premature ejaculation, and the problem is solved. In my book: *Learn to Relax with Meditation*, there is a chapter about Tantra and this will teach you to control your ejaculation.

Premature birth
Reason: To get rid of the child in your body. Or too much stress.
Suppressed Feelings: Pregnancy is too difficult or you don't want to have the baby in your body.
Action: Be aware of your desire to keep the child separate from you.

Prostatitis
Reason: Conflict about your own sexuality; the conflict between being a softy or macho; a conflict between the female and the male side of you. Eating the wrong food; a diet with too much meat, that is too acidic, produces too many toxins in the bowels. Normally the toxins travel downward so that the prostate and sexual organs get all the toxic waste from our food.
Suppressed Feelings:
Action: To express your sexuality without any judgments about what is normal or natural. Detox your body with fasting or do the colon cleaning from Blessed Herbs. Change the food you eat, see the food chapter for more guidance.

Prostatic enlargement.
Reason:
Eating the wrong food; a diet with too much meat, that is too acidic, produces too many toxins in the bowels. Normally the toxins travel downward so that the prostate and sexual organs get all the toxic waste from our food. Learn to let go of your problems; such as your fear of getting older, lose the power; stop being over masculine; stop doing what does not help to fulfill your own goals, focus on the demands for your ideal life.
Suppressed Feelings:
Action: Change the food you eat, see the food chapter for more guidance. Detox your body with fasting or do a colon cleaning with Blessed Herbs. Learn to accept aging and focus on having something fulfilling in your life. As we age, we should integrate our female and male sides. To be macho for your whole life is boring, begin to see and appreciate the female side of yourself.

What is the point of attaining all the high and outstanding goals if we don't enjoy the here and now?

Psoriasis
Reason: The desire to protect yourself with armor against the world in order not to get hurt inside.
Suppressed Feelings: Fear of rejection, getting hurt.
Action: Learn to protect yourself, and then learn to be sensible and open to everybody. If you can't bear your openness then protect yourself.

Pyrosis, heartburn (gastric)
Reason: To hide your aggression so that the anger produces too much acid in the stomach; to swallow anger.
Suppressed Feelings: Anger.
Action: Learn to express your anger.

Rash
Reason: There are many conflicts that we haven't processed, that emerge on the surface. It is a conflict on the border between what happens and what we don't want, like too much intimate contact. On this part of the skin, we get a rash.
Suppressed Feelings: Fear of aggression.
Action: Look at what conflicts are on the border (skin) and like to emerge. For instance, you have a problem saying no when somebody wants to kiss you, but you are not interested in them, then this is a conflict. Or maybe you don't comfortable in your skin. Or you desire intimate contact, and yet you are afraid of intimacy.

Retinal detachment
Reason: 60% short-sightedness, 35% aging, 5% aphakia; flashes, veils, shadows can be the precursor of partial blindness. To have seen too many terrible, and dreadful things in our life that we don't want to see anymore.

Suppressed Feelings: Fear, terror, frightened about specific events.
Action: To release the terrible, frightening situation in our life, so that we can see the things that we have suppressed.

Rheumatism
Reason: Not enough physical exercise. Eating the wrong food, eating food that is too acidic. Old, forgotten problems prevent the progress to move your life forward; communication problems with too little inner flexibility; the stiffness of the joints shows the inflexibility and intransigence to manage life; inhibition of aggression in the consciousness and aggressive attacks against the joints, so that they are painful; the inability to accept your own aggression; not able to solve relationship problems; the patient uses his disease to blackmail his relationships, in order to get compassion from those around him.
Suppressed Feelings:
Action: Changing the food your eat, becoming a vegan or adopting a simple healthy lifestyle, see previous chapters for more information. Fasting is also good. Become more flexible inside and don't blackmail other people. Instead of fighting with the world, go inside yourself and examine your shortcomings. With self-knowledge, you can change and become a better, healthier person inside and out.

Short-sightedness, myopia
Reason: Fear of the future; over intellectual; desire only to see what is nearby with a lack of an overview and looking at the big picture; strong subjectivity because you don't want to see the full picture; resistance to see the world as it is; to neglect the feelings; suppressed fear and anger about your life, so we prefer to read instead of to live; to protect us from the world, we love to see through the glasses the world instead of experiencing it firsthand.
Suppressed Feelings: Fear

Action: To look inside at what we don't want to see. Go to a holistic workshop for learning to see what is all around you and to gain self-knowledge.

Sinusitis general, frontal sinus, maxillary sinus, nasal cavity sinus

Reason: 1. General: Fear of conflicts. 2. Frontal sinus: Little or no intuition. 3. Maxillary sinus: Curbing aggression or suppressed sadness 4. Nasal cavity sinus

Suppressed Feelings:

Action: Over 2 years, I took antibiotics, again and again, every 6 weeks I got sinusitis or a sore throat. Then I stopped the antibiotics, went to encounter groups and now for over 30 years I have never gotten frontal, maxillary sinusitis, or a sore throat again. With the antibiotic, you weaken the immune system so much, that you easily attract the next inflammation. 1. General: Express your feelings. 2. Frontal sinus: Confront yourself with the things and people that you don't like. Fight for your rights. 3. Maxillary sinus: Live your aggression instead of running away from them. 4. Nasal cavity sinus: Confront the good and bad parts of yourself, have the strength and courage to question yourself.

Sore throat

Reason: You don't want to swallow any more problems. It is too much.

Suppressed Feelings: Conflicts

Action: Retreat from the world and look at what you want and what you don't want (so that you don't have to speak), take time to recover, and the next time doesn't swallow everything, you need to better articulate what you want.

Spiritual crises

Reason: A spiritual growth that is too fast, learning about the spiritual world too quickly, so you lose your control over yourself. The risk is to get mad.

Suppressed Feelings:

Action: Grounding through working in the garden, meditation, exhausting sex, cleaning the house, eating heavy food, and trekking in nature with a heavy backpack.

Sterility for men

Reason: Not accepting one's masculinity; you feel that you don't have the confidence/feel worthy to procreate. Eating toxic food, and too many medications.

Suppressed Feelings: Having feelings that you are not a real or good enough spouse who can procreate.

Action: Take responsibility for yourself, and for a child that you desire. See the food chapter for more information.

Stomach diseases

Reason: To swallow too much annoyance. According to Chinese Healing, too much worry; taking life too seriously. Wrong food.

Suppressed Feelings: Desire for your mother's love, needing to get care from your mother.

Action: Process your conflicts with awareness, otherwise the stomach will become too acidic. Open your mouth when something is going against you, don't be the child who chose to be quiet instead of voicing your opinion. Aggression is good if we need to say what we are concerned about. Express your emotions instead of holding them back. If we articulate our problems with a weak voice, nobody understands that something concerns us. See the Qigong element and spleen. Change your food, see food chapter for guidance.

Irritable Stomach

Reason: Unable to digest the impressions you get from the world. Excessive demand to accept life as it is, and to accept the demands on you. This is caused too by eating the wrong food, see the food chapter for more details.

Suppressed Feelings:

Action: Try to solve the problems or let them go. A good area to focus on is to enjoy a stress-free life as much as possible. Change your food, see food chapter for guidance.

Stroke

Reason: The food you eat is too acidic, medications. You have too much stress in your life.
Suppressed Feelings:
Action: Change your lifestyle/food, see chapter food, and focus on prevention. A raw food eater can't get a stroke! Choose stress less/free life.

Snoring

Reason: Too conservative; disturbed contacts with the outside world; like to be alone in the night; not feeling enough respect from others during the day, so that you demand respect during the night, unfortunately, your partner is overwhelmed by the snoring; during the day you spend your time living inside your head (over intellectual), and caring for other people, so then the suppressed anger in the night disturbs everyone else around you.
Suppressed Feelings: You hold deep aggression against other people.
Action: Try the Mp3 for snoring from Dr. Steve G. Jones. Feel your anger during the day and if necessary let it out. Develop ways so you get respect and the dominance that you need during the day.

Tachycardia, fast heartbeat.

Reason: Emotional disorder, feeling torn inside; huge fears; wanting to escape.
Suppressed Feelings: Fear.
Action: Do the things that you want and feel your fears with all aspects. Face your challenges and let yourself feel all of your fears. Make a fear list, with all aspects, prioritize them and then the fears are gone. Listen to the Mp3 Dr. Steve G. Jones, about fears, anxieties.

Tonsillitis

Reason: Have swallowed already too much anger in order to get love and acceptance.
Suppressed Feelings:
Action: To learn to express anger when it is necessary and to protect yourself when it is too much for you.

Tooth root inflammation

Reason: Too much stress
Suppressed Feelings:
Action: The easiest way is to take Colloidal Silver. If this works for your body (doesn't kill the bacteria in the bowels), use it for 14 days or go to the dentist or take antibiotics for 14 days. Afterward, eat raw fermented vegetables daily for 4 weeks.

Thrombosis

Reason: An unhealthy lifestyle. You are eating food that is too acidic, and you are not getting enough physical exercise.
Suppressed Feelings:
Action: See chapters about prevention, and food. Clean your arteries by eating fruits and drinking fresh fruit juices.

Twitching of the limbs.

Reason: Suppressed movements and energy is unloaded, so that twitching begins.
Suppressed Feelings:
Action: Begin dancing freestyle, take up a sport like jogging or the Dynamic Meditation from Osho.

Underactive Thyroid

Reason: To hide yourself behind thick walls; less interest in living; huge disappointments in life; deep frustrations.
Suppressed Feelings: Fear of life.
Action: Go on a retreat in a temple, ashram, or monastery. Confront yourself with the death in your imagination. Find the reason inside of you, the passion for your life.

The mouth of the Uterus cancer
Reason: Unable to protect yourself against sexual attacks.
Suppressed Feelings: Fear of loss of their sexual partner.
Action: Really, learn to say what you want and do not want! This you also need to do in sexual matters with your partner.

Cancer of the uterus
Reason: Never got fulfillment in sex with a man, high frustration in sex life, never enjoyed sex or only had sex out of obligation, have an unfulfilled desire for a child.
Suppressed Feelings:
Action: Go to a body and feelings orientated therapist and work through this cancer. I don't think you can solve the problem alone without a therapist. It is clear that there are some past traumas that caused it.

Inflammation of the vagina
Reason: Unwillingness to have sex with your partner or with men. You are with the wrong partner. Resistance to surrender your love and sex with your mate.
Suppressed Feelings:
Action: Learn to say no and choose the right partner. Learn to surrender and overcome your shame, and fear of sex.

Vaginal mycosis
Reason: Sexuality without love.
Suppressed Feelings: Aggression against yourself and your sex partner.
Action: Enjoy your sexuality and choose the right partner.

Whooping cough, pertussis
Reason: Built-up anger.
Suppressed Feelings: Built-up anger.

Action: Parents need to help their children learn to express their anger in constructive and healthy ways, children need to be taught that anger is necessary to become strong!

The Best Addresses for Holistic Doctors and Clinics

The best Tibetan doctors are in Dharamsala/Himchai Pradesh/India place of the Dalai Lama
Otherwise in Pune:

Dr. Kalsang Tibetan Doctor 6138309. Flat B /5 Ragvilas Society, North Main Road, Koregaon Park, Pune 411001, close to the Ashram of Osho.

Best Ayuveda Doctor is **TriGuna** in Delhi, he opened his clinic in 1933
Vaid Brihaspati Dev Triguna Clinic
No-143, Nizamuddin, Sarai Kale Khan, Delhi - +(91)-11-65165555

Tao Garden
Mantak Chia / Chiang Mai/ Thailand www.tao-garden.com/ This is the best Spa in Thailand, it is internationally renowned. He has all kinds of different alternative treatments, including Ajurveda, Osteopathy, Homeopathy, and Chinese healing.

Scoliosis: There is **Pjotr Elkunoviz** who created a cure for Scoliosis, and he had trained many healers in Germany to do so too. Within seconds your back is straight again. German health insurance pays for it. www.Zfgh.info

Best Books

The Healing Power of Illness: Understanding What Your Symptoms Are Telling You, (Difficult to find) by Thowald Detlefsen (Krankheit als Weg) and Dr. med. Rüdiger Dahlke.

Krankheit als Schlüssel from bestselling Author: Dr. med. Rüdiger Dahlke.

Acupuncture Without Needles, Dr J. V. Cerney

http://www.universal-tao.com/ for books and Cd by Mantak Chia *Awaken Healing, Inner Organ Massage*, Tao - Love…

Healing Your Eyes with Chinese Medicine. Acupuncture, Acupressure &Chinese Herbs, by Andy Rosenfarb

Better Eyesight without Glasses. W. H. Bates, M. D.

Healing Back Pain. The Mind-Body Connection. John E. Sarno, M. D.

The book for Diabetes: There is a Cure for diabetes, from Gabriel Cousens

Reversing Heart Diseases, by Dr. Julian Whitaker M. D.

The Juiceman's Power of juicing. Jay Kordich

Power Juices Super Drinks. Quick, Delicious Recipes to Prevent & Reverse Disease. Steve Meyerowitz

More from the Author

I really hope that I could help you to find inner peace, to enjoy more of your life… Thank you for the reading of my book. I have written four more books in English,

Enjoy your life now!
http://www.amzn.com/B012DFPHJ8 ,

Learn to Relax with Meditation.
https://www.amazon.com/dp/B01561ZWBO ,

Heal yourself and stay healthy!
http://www.amzn.com/B016BJPXXC

The Essence to Become Happy, Healthy and Successful!
http://www.amzn.com/B06XWYL6WF .

The Magic or Qigong.
 http://amzn.com/B0759PJVF8

Why the Religions have failed and not God?
http://amzn.com/B0786TXMR5

 When you click on them, you can see and buy them on Amazon. In the back of this book, you find the description.

I have also created an online Meditation course on YouTube… For free.

Go to my channel, here you find the Meditation course.

(https://www.youtube.com/c/RudiZimmerer)

As a self-publishing author, most of my reviews come directly from readers. It would mean a lot to me if you left a review for this book. Thank you very much for reading my work!

Subscribe to my Newsletter: Relax with Meditation. This is a Newsletter about Spirituality, Psychology, Religion, Health… Here you get two times a week good insights, and you can connect with me and ask a question.

(https://ask-rudy.com/newsletter/)

Have an awesome day

Rudi

PS: If you like to be in my Facebook Group: Relax With Meditation then click here.

(https://www.facebook.com/groups/RelaxWithMeditation/)

If you have an Ipod, connect with my Channel: Relax with Meditation https://itunes.apple.com/us/podcast/relax-with-meditation/id1245179712?mt=2

My other Books:

Enjoy Your Life Now!

How to Become Happy and Successful with powerful techniques from East and West.

1. I have compiled in over 30 years the most efficient techniques to find true happiness and true love.
2. How to change your life in every aspect with feelings and body-orientated therapy combined with meditation.

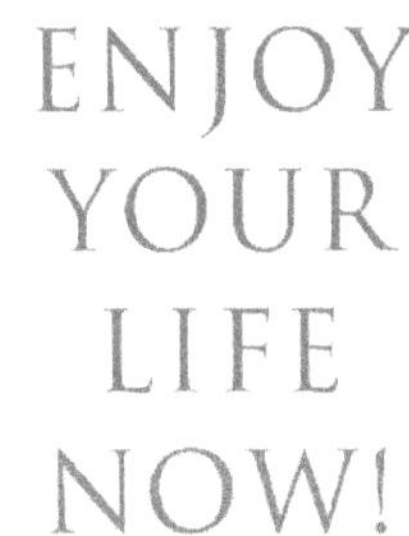
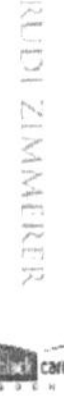
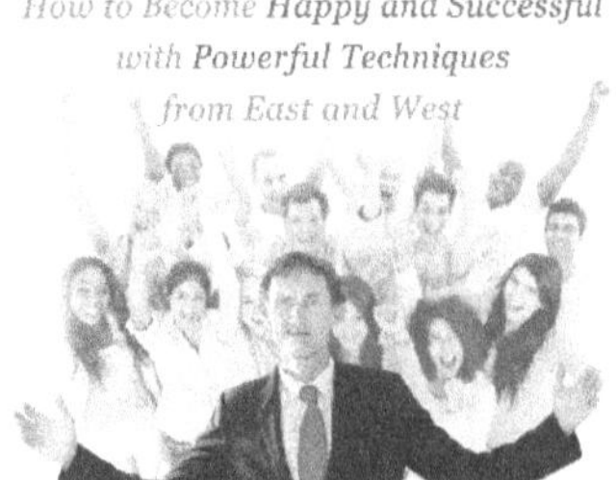

1. **How to get back the love** or connection you may not have received as a child.
2. **How to feel true love** in all your relationships.
3. How to have more fulfilling relationships.
4. How to deal with problems when you are working.
5. **How to live a fulfilled life** even when many things are running against you.
6. Learn that we manifest in our lives what is inside of us regardless if we are aware of it or not.
7. What is true happiness, true love, and true meditation?
8. You will learn the most effective EFT.
9. You will learn why meditation and body exercise is so necessary for living a fulfilled life.
10. And much more you find in my book: Enjoy your life now.

Buy this book from Amazon.
https://amzn.com/B012DFPHJ8

Learn to Relax with Meditation

How to gain Bliss & Inner Peace with the Energy Meditation, Chi Gong, God Love, Tantra, Tao-Love…

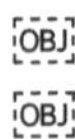

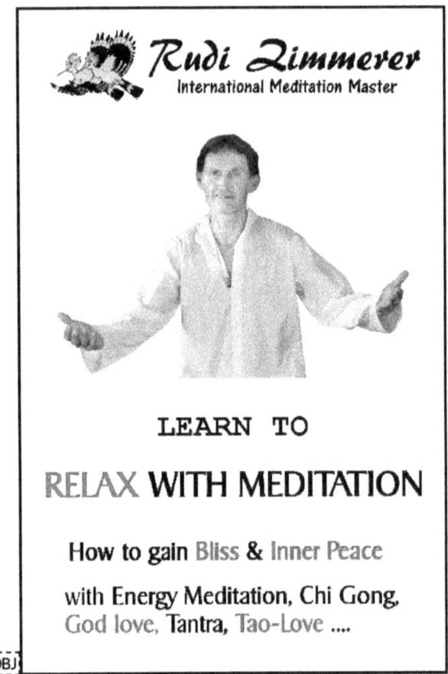

Most people don't understand that meditation reflects what is inside of us. When we are fighting against our thoughts, sometimes we don't even know that our suppressed feelings have caused the thoughts. This book shows:

1. how to release negative emotions with EFT;
2. how to gain bliss with the energy pump;
3. how to ground negative thoughts so that they disappear;

4. how God can benefit our meditation and life;
5. how we can learn to love God;
6. how we can use Tantra and Tao love to gain great results fast for our meditation and spirituality and to enjoy our sexuality;
7. how to achieve health through releasing negative suppressed feelings, the right food, and through the Chi Gong exercises.

Buy this book from *Amazon*.   https://www.amzn.com/B01561ZWBO

The Magic of Qigong!

With the Immortal Qigong,
Fulfilling Bliss and Tao-Love.

Qigong Master Rudi Zimmerer

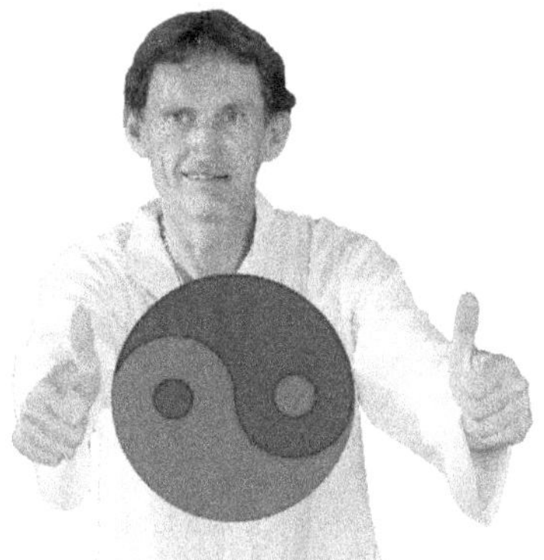

In this book, you will learn the most efficient Qigong. You will discover all the secrets of Qigong that never had been published in one book before. And you need only one hour per day to become healthy and vigor. With the Immortal Qigong is long levity over 100 years possible.

This book teaches you:

1. Do You want to release fast and efficient your negative emotions? With the Tao 5 Elements and the Healing Sounds, you can do so.

2. Do You want to balance your Energy in your body? With Tao Two Hand Method and the Healing Sounds, you can do so.

3. Do You want Peace in your mind and experience Bliss? With my moving Qigong, you will gain that and excellent Health.

4. Do You want to Live Long and to be Healthy and Vigor? With the Immortal Qigong from Lu Zijian (Lu Zijian died with 118 and was vigor and healthy until his end), you achieve that, and you will get Bliss and Peace in mind.

5. Do You want to Enjoy Your Sex, to have a longer Climax and even to Heal our body? With the Tao-Love, you do so.

6. Do you have problems to learn new things? You can easily learn my Qigong with my videos. For free, You can download and see my Qigong videos.

Buy this book from Amazon . http://amzn.com/B0759PJVF8

The Essence to Become Happy, Healthy and Successful!

From my Facebook Group: Relax with Meditation

In this book, I include the best for our happiness, health, success and spirituality in easily consumable portions from my Facebook Group: Relax with Meditation. There are 140 articles quick to read and to understand. Just open the book somewhere, read one article, relax and improve your life. You don't have to read the whole book, just one article at a time ... is enough. I found a great article from the very successful Man Dr. Patrick Liew (Co-Founder Success Resources), "How to re-craft our life?" I asked him, to use this material for my book, and he also wrote the foreword.

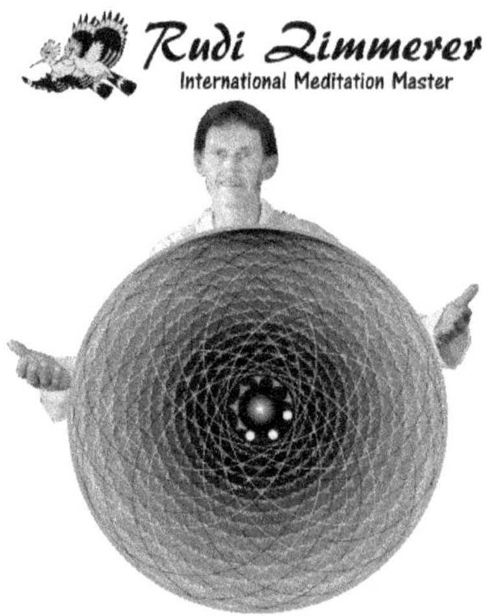

In my book I describe:

1. Why we don't get what we want?

2. How to Overcome Procrastination?

3. What is an optimal time management?

4. How to get our life back?

5. How to get rid of our Anger?

6. How to become creative?

7. How to improve our relationships?

8. How to become Forever Young?

9. What is the best for our Immune system!

10. What are the causes of all diseases and the cure?

11. How to cure cancer?

12. What is the meaning of our life?

13. Is there more?

14. What is God?

15. Why is it so important to have a God relationship?

16. I can't die, I am Energy… ?

17. Is There A Free Will?

18. Fake Gurus - True Gurus?

Buy this book from Amazon

http://www.amzn.com/B06XWYL6WF

Why the Religions have failed and not God?

Why don't exist Hell, Paradise, Moksha, Nirvana and Enlightenment?

This book is written for people who are frustrated from the Organized Religions and the spiritual Masters. People who like to connect with God and don't like to obey stupid rules of the Religions.

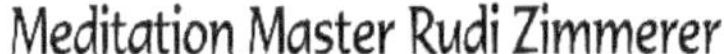

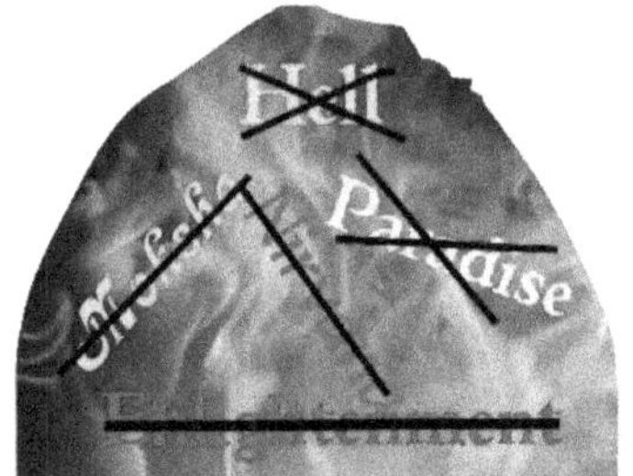

You will learn:

1. That the organized Religions are just another Spam!

2. Why don't exist Paradise and Hell?

3. Why don't exist Nirvana, Moksha, and Enlightenment?

4. It doesn't exist a final death -science proofed by the Research done on 996 people.

5. The worst and cruelest verses of the Quran and the Bible.

6. The Quran encourages to enslave, kill, rape and torture Nonbelievers of the Islam.

7. What is God?

8. How important is it to have a personal God relationship?

9. How to connect to God?

10.   That sex is good and healthy.

Buy this book from Amazon http://amzn.com/B0786TXMR5

Give your life a meaning or enjoy…

Consider please:

Nothing has a meaning until we give it a meaning.

If we would enjoy our entire life, we don't need a meaning for our life.

Most people can't enjoy their life even they can't enjoy their working time… I will help you in this book to enjoy your entire life!

Still, we should give our life a meaning that will direct our life. So that we know why we do this and not waste our time for meaningless things…

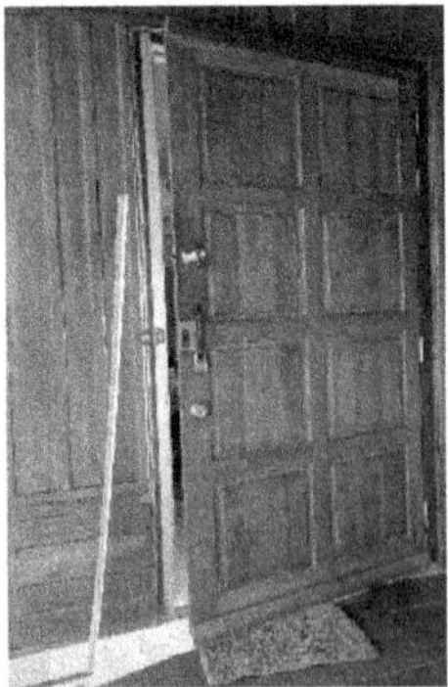

You find the answers in this book.

1. Why can't we enjoy our life?

2. Why are good relationships more important than wealth and success?

3. Why should we care for our intimacy relationships?

4. Why do we need to enjoy our Job?

5. Why do we need a goal setting?

6. Why can't we rely on our kids as the meaning of life?

7. Why should we fulfill our heart desires?

8. Why is it essential to have a mission?

9. Why should we stop regretting instead to do it?

10.   Why should we learn to go beyond our desires?

11.   Why do we need to be connected with God/divine?

12.   Why can God/Divine give us a meaning of life?

Buy this book from Amazon   https://www.amzn.com/B07NLM3MS9

My healing center

Within the next five years, I want to create a healing center with the best alternative doctors and therapists. My idea is that every patient will have a coach and therapist:

1. To find the (psychosomatic) reason for the diseases.
2. To find a life mission, a reason to live for patients with severe diseases.
3. To open up the heart and the feelings.
4. To release the fear of failure to help in healing the disease.
5. To give the patients the faith that their disease will be cured.
6. To help to create a more fulfilling life after the cure.

I want to offer:

- Tibetan doctor for herbs and acupuncture
- Chinese doctor TCM,
- Homeopathy,
- Ayurveda,
- Osteopathy
- Massage
- Recreation, swimming pool, gymnastic room, Chi Gong, and yoga

In India, we can find the best alternative doctors and also the cheapest treatments. Therefore, I think a place close to the ocean between Madras and Pondicherry would be great. The price for one square foot costs between 100 and 300Indian Rs (USD1.5 and USD4.5).
Or another idea is just to open this healing center in a good hotel, where people can come and have the treatment and stay.

Learn The Cause Of Diseases And How To Heal Diabetes, Cancer, Heart, Back...

I have written this book, because of so many wrong concepts for healing the body... I want to help you, to get your health back, in easily doable steps and as fast as possible. I want that you enjoy your life because I know how hard it is to suffer from diseases, to lose all of our hopes.

Do you want to heal your heart, cancer, your back, diabetes and 140 other diseases? Then this book is for you. Even more, I describe how to live a healthy life with good food, body exercise, and Qigong. I describe the best Qigong exercises and give you the best addresses or links for healing that I have found in this book.

Before you heal your body heal first your soul.

The cause of diseases are suppressed feelings, stress, unhealthy food, western medicaments, too less exercise, too less sleep and rest.

1. Why we treat our body so bad with unhealthy food, overeating, not enough exercise, too much stress...?
2. Why is faith the most important thing in our healing?
3. Why is fear or no faith in the healing the worst?
4. Why can't Western medicine give us health and weakens our body?
5. Why we need a healthy lifestyle, with healthy food such as fresh juices, sprouts, green smoothies and time for rest, relaxation and body exercise?